# Fit and Proud

## A Gay Man's Guide to Fitness and Well-Being After 55

**Aiden Hunter**

# Table of Contents

# Introduction

Everyone wants to live a long, healthy life. That much is true. However, that doesn't mean everyone enjoys aging. Let's be honest: No one likes getting older, and understandably so. As we age, our health typically starts deteriorating. Our bodies become weaker, and over time, we become unable to do the things we used to be able to do without breaking a sweat. On top of that, our bodies change physically as well as perceptibly. Wrinkles appear all over the place, we endure having to watch our hair fall away, and various parts of our bodies start to sag... That's not exactly pleasant, especially considering the "young is beautiful" concept that's shoved down our throats at every turn. No matter what some people may say, ageism is a thing that exists, and not getting upset at the fact that you are getting older can be rather difficult at times.

Now, you can't exactly stop the aging process, at least not unless you have some sort of time machine—in which case, do share! Since you can't stop aging, you have to do two things instead. First, you must accept that aging is part of life. You even have to embrace and find the beauty within aging. Before you object: Yes, beauty within aging exists. Second, you must figure out how to age while remaining as strong, independent, mobile, and healthy as humanly possible. You see, contrary to what many people think, aging doesn't have to mean becoming irrelevant, incapable, or anything of the sort. You can, in fact, remain perfectly strong, capable of doing many of the things you used to do as a youngster at 50, 60, and beyond. You just need to know what steps to take to make that possible and then actually take those steps.

Yeah, so what are those steps? The surface-level answer to that question is "working out and eating healthy." However, the actual steps you need to take to age well while maintaining your strength, mobility, and independence are a little more complicated. For example, consider the following questions:

- Are there any exercises that men should do, especially once they've hit 55? If so, what are they, and how do you do them?

- Are there any exercises men over 55 should avoid, for that matter? Why?

- How often should I actually be working out, and for how long? How intense should my workouts be?

- Is there anything I really should be eating at 55 to ensure that my aging mind and body get all the nutrients they need? Are there any food items that I really should try to keep out of my diet?

- How about mental health? Given the stigma that the LGBTQ+ community has faced all their lives, are there any mental health concerns I should especially be aware of at 55? If so, what can I do to avoid them and improve my mental health?

- Is there anything I should do for sexual health, given that I'm not a celibate monk, even if I am 55 and most of the world seems to expect people to become celibate monks after they reach a certain age?

These are just some examples of the questions you must consider as you age. They're also examples of the kinds of questions we will be answering throughout the course of *Fit and Proud*. This book is written for the exact purpose of helping gay men over the age of 50, such as myself, figure out how to be the fittest, healthiest, strongest, and happiest version of themselves as they age and at any age. It's written for readers who, like me, acknowledge that aging is a part of natural life and want to make their later years in life as comfortable, independent, active, and fabulous as possible. If that sounds like the kind of life you want to lead in your 50s and beyond, then this book is for you. The following chapters contain all the secrets you need to live the life you desire—you just need to turn the page.

# Chapter 1:

# Understanding the Aging Process

We all want to stay young. We all want to look young. Who can blame us? Especially when there are massive industries focused on helping us look younger than we actually are. No matter how big the plastic surgery and skincare industries are and how great their procedures and products are, we all age. That is inevitable. However, aging doesn't have to be the ugly, catastrophic life event that Hollywood makes it out to be. It doesn't have to mean being confined to your home, unable to do half the things you used to be able to do for the creaking of your bones. Instead, aging can be a graceful process, one where your body goes through certain changes—there's no getting around that—without limiting you or causing your quality of life to drop.

For this future to be possible, though, there are specific things you need to do. You need to take certain precautions in your daily life. You have to look out for your body by feeding it the right food and doing the right exercises. What does the term "right" mean, though? To answer that question, we have to understand exactly what kind of changes our bodies go through as we age. By that, I don't just mean our hair graying and our faces getting wrinkled. Those are issues we can take care of with a little bit of hair dye—assuming we don't want to pull off the silver fox look—and Botox. Instead, I mean our metabolism, which slows down as we age, making it difficult for us to maintain our fit and fabulous figure. I mean the loss of muscle mass and bone density that happens with aging, too. So, without further ado, let's take a look at exactly what these changes mean for us and, more importantly, how we can manage them.

# How the Body Changes With Age

To understand what happens to our body as we age, we must first understand what happens to our cells. Our cells are the components of our bodies. They knit together our tissues, organs, and skin. Our cells aren't immortal. They age, and after a certain point, they die. Their lifespans are relatively short, though. So, when cells do die, newer, younger models take their place. Here's the thing: Our cells cannot keep dying and getting replaced by their newer "trophy wife" models indefinitely. After a certain point, they lose this ability. This point is when aging truly begins. It's when our skin starts wrinkling, our hair starts whitening, and other similar changes start happening in our various organs and systems (Nazario, 2023).

Take your brain as an example. Did you know that as you age, your brain starts getting smaller and smaller? This process starts when you hit your 30s and 40s. However, it really picks up speed when you're in your 60s. As your brain gets smaller, it starts getting less blood and, therefore, less oxygen, too. At the same time, the connections between your brain cells, meaning your neurons, weaken. As time goes on and these effects start building up, you start noticing their consequences. For example, you are very forgetful. You leave your keys somewhere and forget where you've put them. You draw a blank when you're trying to remember the word for something or maybe even forget someone's name for a moment. For your sake, I hope that someone isn't your partner and that you don't slip up and call him your ex's name—because that's a can of worms you just don't want to open. Believe me.

Forgetfulness isn't the only side effect of this situation. Another symptom is trouble concentrating. You see, as we age, our attention span keeps shrinking as our brains do. So, we become less able to focus on things for extended periods of time. Learning new things, like a new language, become harder (but not impossible).

Meanwhile, your heart and cardiovascular system start undergoing some changes as well. For instance, as you age, your blood vessels become harder and thicker, just like... Well, you get the joke. However, this process is a bit problematic because as vessels lose their elasticity, your circulation slows down because your heart and vessels have a harder time pushing blood onward. As you near your 60s, you start losing what doctors call "pacemaker" cells. These are cells that basically tell your heart to beat. As you lose your pacemaker cells, your heart slows down, at least compared to when you were 25.

This situation isn't necessarily problematic, but it can be if you're not careful. After all, there's a reason why a lot of people have heart trouble. That doesn't mean everyone who ages ends up with heart trouble, of course. It just means that exercising, being active, and eating well become doubly important for keeping your heart and cardiovascular system healthy.

How are your senses? Well, there's no question that all your senses start declining as you age, except perhaps your gaydar. Your vision, for example, starts declining. It's not uncommon for someone to experience things like blurry vision and other eye problems from their 40s onward. It's also not uncommon for colors to look less vibrant to you. A similar kind of thing happens with your ears. As you age, hearing can become more and more difficult. Currently, about half of the population experiences age-related hearing loss to some degree by the time they turn 75 (*Age-Related Hearing Loss (Presbycusis*, 2015).

What about taste? Well, something very interesting happens with your sense of taste right around when you hit your 50s: certain flavors start tasting differently for you. Foods that you used to enjoy turn a bit more bland or bitter. Things that used to be very salty or sweet feel less so. A similar change happens with your sense of smell, with your nose becoming less and less sensitive to scents.

A comparable thing happens with your sense of touch as your skin loses nerve endings. Your skin also starts producing less elastin and collagen. Because of this decline, you get wrinkles and your skin starts to sag in certain places. Less elastin and collagen also mean you bruise more easily and take longer to heal. Becoming overheated becomes far too easy as you age, and not just because you're so hot.

## Your Metabolism, Muscle Mass, and Bone Density

One of the biggest complaints that aging people tend to have is that they can't do the same things that they used to do. For example, they can't eat the quantity of food they used to eat and still stay in shape. They can't run as fast as they used to or move about as quickly. They don't feel as strong either, and they have a harder time performing everyday tasks than they used to, like lifting things or reaching for a high shelf.

So, why do these things happen? The answer to that question lies in your metabolism, muscle mass, and bone density. To start, let's take a look at your metabolism. Your metabolism is the catch-all term for the chemical processes that happen inside your body to keep it functioning. Without being too technical, or rather biological, about it, your metabolism unfolds in two phases. Phase one happens when your body breaks down the nutrients you consume and turns them into energy for you to use. Phase two happens when you use the molecules that your body creates by breaking down those nutrients to create other useful substances like muscle protein to build muscle.

Here's the issue: As you age, your metabolism slows down. In essence, it loses its ability to break down nutrients quickly. As a result, those nutrients, like glucose, hang out in your system and bloodstream for longer. This process causes your blood sugar levels and the like to spike more quickly. At the same time, nutrients get stored in your body instead of broken down. This process is what happens with fat, for example, which is why losing weight becomes harder as you age.

Simultaneously, your body loses its ability to create things like muscle protein. Hence, its ability to build muscle slowly goes down. Not only that but once you hit 50, your body actually starts losing 0.4 pounds of muscle mass annually. A similar occurrence happens with your bones. As you age, you lose bone mass. Your bones become less dense and more brittle, making it far easier for you to break an arm or hip when you fall, for example.

There's good news, though: This outcome doesn't have to be the case. In fact, you actually have the power to speed up your metabolism and prevent muscle mass and bone density loss. You just need to exercise a little and eat well, as you'll see in the coming chapters.

As with anything even remotely medical, the muscle mass loss that comes with age has a complicated-sounding name: sarcopenia. If you are physically inactive and over the age of 30, you will have lost 3–5% of your muscle mass by the time you're 40 (Ambardekar, 2022). As you keep aging, you'll lose even more than that. Over time, the effects of this loss will build up. So, you'll start feeling weaker than you used to. You'll lose a bit of your stamina, too. This loss will mainly occur because your body won't be able to produce as much muscle protein as it used to, but scientists believe there are also other reasons for it. For example, remember how you start losing nerve cells as you age? Well, as a result, you end up with fewer cells sending signals to your muscles, telling them to move. At the same time, you start producing less testosterone. Since testosterone plays a part in muscle development, muscle shrinkage is also a result.

How about bone density loss, then? You see, your bones regularly undergo two processes without you even realizing it: bone breakdown and bone formation. Both processes are perfectly natural. Before the age of 25, your bone formation process outpaces your bone breakdown process, so much so that the former could run laps around the latter. When you turn 25, your bone formation process slows down a bit, and it starts keeping pace with the bone breakdown process. This pacing continues until you turn 50 (*Osteoporosis: What You Need to Know as You Age*, n.d.). Then, things change once again, and your bone production process slows down even more. Thus, like the tort going up against the hare, your bone breakdown process takes the lead, and bit by bit, you start losing bone density. So, you start feeling a little weaker once again, and your bones get a little more brittle with the passage of time, too.

Again, though, this outcome doesn't have to be the case. In fact, there are many things you can do and lots of different exercises you can work into your daily life to keep muscle mass and bone density loss at bay. When added to your routine, some activities will strengthen your bones and muscles so that you remain fit, strong, and healthy for years to come. Before we dive into what those activities and exercises are, though, let's take a quick look at one last thing: the common health issues that you, as a gay man, might find yourself dealing with once you've hit 55.

## Common Health Issues for Gay Men Over 55

First, let's get the most obvious thing out of the way: HIV. HIV is a scary disease, especially if you've already witnessed how devastating it can be. However, these days, HIV is not the death sentence it used to be. It's a very manageable disease. Thanks to the wonder of modern science, current HIV medication can help anyone who has been diagnosed with HIV to live a long and healthy life and keep them from transmitting the disease to others.

Just as there are anti-HIV meds you can take, there are also ones that prevent HIV. These medications are called pre-exposure prophylaxis (PrEP), and they can eliminate your chances of catching HIV. Of course, that doesn't mean you should have unprotected sex, especially if you have more than one partner—something you probably learned in your wild, glorious youth. If you are exposed, taking PrEP within 72 hours of exposure will help, as you probably already know. My advice in this case, though, is to know where you can get PrEP in advance. To my mind, this is one of those cases where the boring saying "Better safe than sorry" proves true (*10 Things Gay Men Should Discuss*, n.d.).

Cancer is another thing you might want to keep in mind as you age. Specifically, prostate, colon, and testicular cancers are the types that men, especially gay men, may be at risk of. A great way to mitigate this risk is to get regular screenings at least once a year. You'll want to keep your fun bits fun and safe no matter what age you are, after all.

Speaking of checkups, they need to become a regular part of your life as you grow older and wiser—for your eyes, ears, and teeth as well. Studies show that two percent of all gay men experience visual impairment as they age. They also show that 20% of them experience hearing loss. Meanwhile, nearly a quarter of the LGBT community encounters dental problems with age. About 22% of gay men most certainly do, requiring frequent visits to the dentist (Fredriksen-Goldsen, 2011). With those facts in mind, making regular trips to the doctor and the dreaded dentist can only ever be a good thing, don't you think?

# Chapter 2:

# Setting Fitness Goals

If muscle mass and bone density loss are normal (but annoying) parts of aging, what are we supposed to do? How are we supposed to stay strong, fit, and fabulous? The short answer to that question is "exercise." What kind of exercise, though? That's the question. Are there any specific exercises you should do as you age? How long are you supposed to work out per week? How long are you supposed to work out per day?

Suppose that you used to work out a lot in your twenties. You'd hit the gym and do some very high-intensity exercises. However, over the years, you've dropped out of the habit. You still look fine, fit, and fabulous but are perhaps a bit pudgier than you used to be. Now that you're in your 50s, you recognize that you have to start working out again. You start hitting the gym and trying to get back into your old routine. You quickly realize, however, that things aren't the same as they used to be. You get winded a lot more rapidly than you used to and can't lift the weights that used to be easy.

As disheartening as this situation might feel, it is only to be expected, especially if you haven't worked out in a while. I mean, not only have you lost some muscle mass and bone density over the years, but your conditioning level has gone down. So, raising your conditioning and increasing your strength is going to require time and effort. You won't be able to pick things up where you left off. Instead, you will have to start from your current level and go from there. Granted, you're probably not going to get into the same shape you were when you were 20. If only that were possible! Your body also won't be able to handle the same kind of high-impact workouts as back then. However, that doesn't mean you won't be able to get back into shape. It also doesn't mean you won't regain much strength in your muscles and bones.

# Determining Your Fitness Level

Now, there are two things you have to do before you actually start hitting the gym and working out: You have to determine what your current fitness level is, and, based on that level, you have to set motivating yet achievable and realistic fitness goals for yourself. Determining your fitness level is important because otherwise, you might choose the wrong fitness goals for yourself. The wrong fitness goals aren't just goals that are too hard for you to meet in your current physical state. They can be goals that are too easy for you to meet, meaning they're below your current fitness level.

Before we get started with how you can determine your fitness level, let's first understand what we mean by "fit." When I use the term "fit," I don't just mean it to imply that someone's looking good (Asp, 2024). I use it to imply that someone has the muscle strength, joint flexibility, endurance, and conditioning necessary to perform various physical activities without getting really tired or putting a lot of stress on their body. As a rule, I believe that it's important to stay fit as you age because someone who's truly fit can be as healthy as someone who's about 15 years younger than them.

Trying to determine your fitness levels means taking a fitness test. This fitness test will typically evaluate you in four key areas:

1. Body composition

2. Aerobic fitness

3. Muscle strength and endurance

4. Flexibility

Body composition refers to how much muscle, fat, and bone there is in your body. In other words, it refers to what your body is made of. Aerobic fitness means your heart's ability to use the oxygen you breathe in properly and efficiently. Muscle strength and endurance refer to how hard and for how long your muscles are able to actively work. Finally, there's flexibility, which means well your joints can maintain their full, intended range of motion.

You can assess your fitness level by having a fitness professional, such as a trainer, give you a fitness test. The first thing a trainer will look at in this test is your body composition. They can evaluate this information by determining your body mass index (BMI). BMI is basically a scale that tells you whether you have a healthy amount of fat—yes, there is such a thing—in your body. The way to calculate it is pretty simple, as there is a formula to it:

- (Your current weight in pounds x your height in inches squared) x 703

By following this simple equation, you'll find a number representing your BMI. You'll then be able to take a look at the BMI scale. When you do, you'll come across information that looks like this, at least for adults (Mayo Clinic Staff, 2017):

- **Below 18.5:** You are underweight for your age.

- **Between 18.5 and 24.9:** You are at a normal weight for your age.

- **Between 25.0 and 29.9:** You are overweight for your age.

- **Over 29.9:** You are obese for your age.

Once you've determined your BMI and figured out what it means, you'll move on to the second part of the body composition test. This portion will measure the circumference, that is to say, the size of your waist. Generally, you want your waist to be smaller than your hips. Having a waist that's bigger than your hips is a sign that you might be at risk for type 2 diabetes and heart disease. So, as a man, that means you want your waist size to be smaller than 40 inches.

After you've measured your waist, you can move on to your aerobic test. This test will aim to test and measure your heart health. As an adult, you want your heart rate to be between 60 and 100 beats per minute. To start, the trainer or test-giver you've gone to will take a look at your pulse for 15 seconds. Then, they'll multiply the result they've obtained by four to figure out how many times your heart beats per minute.

Next, they'll strive to measure your target heart zone. Your target heart zone is a measurement of how much your heart beats when you're giving it and the rest of your body a solid workout. For a healthy adult, this zone must be somewhere between 50–70% of their maximum heart rate (MHR) when they're doing moderate-intensity exercises. However, this figure should be about 70–85% of their MHR when they're doing really intense ones.

If this process sounds a little complicated, fear not! I have actual figures I can share with you, too. Take your target heart zone, for example. What does this figure have to be for you to be aerobically fit? For someone who's 55 years old, it must be between 83 and 140 beats per minute. What about your MHR? Again, if you're 55 or thereabouts, it needs to be 165 beats per minute.

Following your aerobic test, you'll undergo your muscle strength and endurance test. Usually, this test will require you to do some push-ups, which you can do on your knees if they're a bit too difficult for you for the moment. As a man, the number of push-ups you should be able to do to be considered fit is a little different from the number of push-ups a woman your age is supposed to be able to do. Women who are 55 should be able to do 10 push-ups in a row, but a 55-year-old man should be able to do 12 in one go.

The final part of your fitness test will gauge your flexibility. You'll have to perform some basic stretches for this test and see how well you do. Some stretches you'll be asked to try out at this stage of the test include these examples (Achauer, 2022):

- **Toe touches:** You have to be able to touch your toes while keeping your legs straight, as this will mean your hips, hamstrings, and back are flexible.

- **Neck twists:** You must sit down on a chair or similar surface and turn your head to one side and the other to see if you can get your chin in line with your shoulder at about a 90-degree angle, indicating that it is indeed flexible.

- **The open book stretch:** You must lie down on a firm surface with your knees bent. You then stretch out both arms in front of you before slowly moving the top one to your other side, where you'll have it touch the floor without moving your legs, pelvis, or other arm, indicating you have spinal flexibility.

# Identifying Your Fitness Goals and Aspirations

Now that you've figured out your fitness level, you can start setting appropriate fitness goals for yourself. By this point, you might be wondering, *Why do I need to set goals? Why can't I just start working out?* Well, consider this scenario: Have you ever started working out, kept at it for a few weeks, then dropped the habit completely because of [insert any excuse here]? I know that I have. I also know that I probably wouldn't have if I'd set fitness goals for myself. You see, goals, by their nature, are very motivating, especially as you meet them. They can ensure you remain committed to working out, staying healthy, and getting fit. That's not all. Fitness goals can make it easier for you to incorporate more physical activity and different exercises into your daily life. They help you spot obstacles to your workouts early on and solve them before they become actual problems. They can make it easy for you to plan your day since setting goals means knowing exactly what you'll be doing and how long it'll take (Lennon, 2020).

That's another thing: Setting fitness goals leaves no doubt in your mind as to what you should be doing when you start your exercise routine. There's no moment of confusion where you're trying to decide whether you should do push-ups or cycling or something else. Your goals tell you what you need to get done so you get to them. It's as simple as that. At least, it will be as simple as that if you know how to set fitness goals because, yes, there is a method to the madness.

So, what are good fitness goals for 55-year-olds, and how do you set them? First, let's start with the basics. Most doctors recommend that you exercise a total of 150 minutes per week, doing moderate-intensity aerobic exercises, or that you exercise a total of 75 minutes of high-intensity aerobic exercises per week. Obviously, that doesn't mean you have to work out for 150 or 75 minutes straight. Instead, you can break up that time into increments of your own choosing. For example, if you decide to exercise five days a week for a total of 150 minutes, then you can do one 30–minute exercise per day. Alternatively, you can plan a schedule like this one (Kendrick, 2023):

- Monday: 30 minutes of exercise

- Tuesday: 20 Minutes of exercise

- Wednesday: 40 minutes of exercise

- Thursday: 30 minutes of exercise

- Friday: 30 minutes of exercise

You can try any other combination you'd like, and you can make use of your weekends. Basically, how you break up your total workout time is up to you, so long as you stick with the recommended workout times.

*Why is this important? I thought we were going to talk about fitness goals.* Knowing how much you have to work out and how you can portion out time throughout the week is important because you don't want to set vague, hard-to-meet fitness goals for yourself. Instead, you want to set SMART fitness goals. The letters in "SMART" represent these strategies (*How to Work out Smarter, Not Harder*, 2022):

- specific

- measurable

- achievable

- relevant

- time-bound

You want the fitness goals you set for yourself to be *specific* because that makes them easier to achieve. Imagine you have a date, and your partner told you to dress nice because where they're taking you is a surprise—only they forgot to tell you whether you should dress casual nice, formal nice, or something else. How hard will it be to pick an outfit? How much will you stress about this decision, and how many different outfits are you going to try in the process?

Just as specificity is important when planning a date, it's important when setting fitness goals. Without specificity, you'll have no clear idea about what you want to achieve and do in a workout session. So, you risk fumbling around and going from one exercise to another, unsure what to do next. If you make your goals specific, though, then you'll know exactly what you need to do to meet them. You'll be able to make the most of your workout time, too.

What about setting *measurable* goals? Fitness goals must be measurable because that makes it possible for you to track your progress. Indeed, specificity and measurability go hand in hand. Here's an example: Which fitness goal do you think is more measurable?

- do more push-ups by the end of the week

- do at least 40 push-ups by the end of the week

Clearly, the latter goal is more measurable. However, this doesn't mean that is the right goal for you. After all, your goals need to be *achievable*, and whether they're achievable or not depends on your current fitness level. That's why you had a fitness test done, remember? If that fitness test showed that you can do 20 push-ups in a row, then aiming for 40 right out the gate isn't going to be doable. But 25 might be possible if you work out regularly, as you should.

What about *relevant* goals? Relevant goals are ones that will help you to achieve the results you want. Say that you want to lose weight, and that's why you started working out again. If that's the case, then goals that are all about weightlifting and muscle-building won't help you achieve weight loss, but goals that involve cardio will. Put another way, weightlifting goals won't be relevant to your fitness aspirations, but aerobic ones will be.

Last but not least, what does it mean for a goal to be *time-bound*? A time-bound goal is one you must complete in a specific amount of time. "Do at least 40 push-ups by the end of the week" is a time-bound goal. "Do more push-ups" isn't. Your fitness goals should be time-bound for two reasons. The first reason is that this strategy makes them more specific and, therefore, easier to meet. The second reason is that time-bound goals make it easy for you to track your progress.

## Creating A Sustainable and Trackable Fitness Plan

Setting SMART fitness goals for yourself is clearly very important if you want to be fit and fabulous. However, as you're setting them, you must remember that you need to have two types of goals: long-term and short-term. Your long-term goals are your fitness aspirations. They're the reason "why" you're working out, be it to lose weight, strengthen your muscles, improve your balance and flexibility, or do something else entirely. Your short-term goals are the goals you'll meet daily, weekly, and monthly to achieve that larger aspiration. More importantly, once you've set your goals, you must create a sustainable and trackable fitness plan.

Step one in creating your fitness plan is determining your fitness level and then setting all your fitness goals. Start the goal-setting process with your largest, most long-term one. Now, start thinking on a smaller scale. What monthly goals can you set for yourself to meet this larger one? What weekly goals can you set to meet the monthly ones? What daily ones can you set to meet the weekly ones? Consider these factors carefully.

Next, decide how intense you want your workouts to be and, consequently, how long they're going to last. Based on that information, decide how many days out of the week you'll be working out. Say that you've decided to do moderate-intensity exercises for 150 minutes per week. How do you want to divide that time? How long do you want your workout sessions to be? Most people keep their workout time to around 30 minutes, but you can do your own thing as long as you meet the 150-hour requirement. As you're dividing up your workout time, though, you should also consider your recovery time.

Recovery time is the rest period you take between bouts of physical activity. This includes both rests you take while working out and the rest days you fit in between your workout days. You might think, *Rest? Who needs rest?* Well, you do, or at least your body does. Here's the thing: When you exercise, you create micro-tears in your muscles. These micro tears then repair themselves and throw in some additional muscle fibers on top of the ones that had existed before—the way one might throw in some extra tip for that hot bartender working his tail off. The problem is that this process doesn't happen immediately. Instead, it takes time, and the best way for you to give your body that time is to knit together those new muscles. The way that one friend might knit you a sweater is to take your rest days.

Clearly, rest days need to be a part of your workout schedule. This is especially true for people over 50 because your muscles' ability to repair themselves slows down as you age. Hence, men over 50 need more recovery time than those in their 20s, and understandably so. There's also the fact that without recovery days, you'll end up getting sick and tired of constantly working out. So, you'll be a lot more likely to quit.

With all that information in mind, here's the obvious question we need to ask: How long should your recovery periods be, and when should you take them? For men over 50 years old, taking two or three recovery days a week is a good idea. These rest days will help them build back their muscles more easily. The same can be said for taking small breaks between workout sets. As a rule, you should take 30- to 60-second long breaks between your sets, depending on how winded you've become (Editors of Men's Health, 2021). You should never sit still during these short breaks. Instead, you should move about and hydrate. By hydrating, I mean to drink water, not iced coffee—as tempting as that might be. By keeping mobile during your breaks, you can bring your heart rate down more slowly, which will be better for your heart health. Speaking of being mobile, you should also make a point of keeping active on your rest days. In other words, you shouldn't be a couch potato these days, at least not all day long. Instead, you should go for a walk, meet with friends, and keep active in general. This will both help with the muscle soreness you'll experience and prove a more pleasant way to spend your time.

So, you've decided which days are going to be your workout and rest days. You've also decided on how long your workout sessions and breaks will be. Now, you have to actually determine what exercises you're going to do during your workouts. Which exercises you're going to do will depend on your answers to two questions:

1. What is your overall workout goal?

2. What, if any, physical limitations are you working with?

Suppose that your overall workout goal is to lose weight. If so, then the exercises you're going to choose will be more cardio-focused. Alternatively, say that your overall goal is to build and strengthen your muscles or to improve your balance and flexibility. For the former, you're going to have to opt for strength training exercises. For the latter, you'll need flexibility and balanced, focused exercises, such as tai chi or yoga.

You'll also need to consider your physical limitations if you have any. Say that you have a bad knee. If that's the case, running or jogging probably won't be the best activity type for you. Neither will any exercise that has you kneeling on the floor, at least not without some padding.

There's one last factor you need to consider as you're putting together your workout schedule: your lifestyle. In other words, how busy you are. Some people lead very busy, even hectic lifestyles that are filled with work, all sorts of social activities, or both. Others lead more relaxed, meditative lifestyles. Both are perfectly alright. You need to know what kind of lifestyle you lead, though, if you want to create a workout schedule that works for you. For example, if you lead a very hectic lifestyle, then scheduling a 30 to 40-minute workout in the day is going to be challenging for you. Scheduling a 10 to 20-minute one, however, might not be. That's perfectly okay. After all, you don't have to work for 30 minutes straight. You just have to get in your 150 or 75 minutes of activity a week, depending on how hard your workout will be.

# *Tracking Progress and Celebrating Milestones*

Creating a fitness schedule that works for you and your lifestyle is very important. Otherwise, making excuses as to why you can't work out right now would be far too easy. I mean, there's a reason why one of the most common excuses for why people don't work out is, "I don't have the time." Creating a workout schedule cuts such excuses off at the knees. It also makes it infinitely easier for you to track your progress and celebrate your milestones.

Wait, why is that important? Can't you just work out regularly and call it a day? You could, but then you'd be missing out. You see, tracking your fitness progress can be immensely motivating, especially if you are new to working out or haven't been working out for a long while when you first started. When you track your fitness progress, you witness firsthand how far you've come. You get to quiet those negative thoughts that can sometimes pop up, like annoying commentators throwing shade and remarking that you haven't been able to advance so much as a single step. After all, you'll be able to show those inner commentators just how many steps you have taken.

Tracking your progress isn't just good for motivation, though. It's something that can hold you accountable. Not everyone enjoys working out all that much, and even those who do sometimes want to skip a workout or two (Brixius, 2022). The problem is that once you skip one, you want to skip the next one and then the next one. Before you know it, you've replaced your daily workouts with more time spent on the couch, watching *Queer Eye* and *America's Next Top Model*, or whatever else takes your fancy. When you track your progress, though, you keep reminding yourself of your goals and all the time and effort you put into meeting them. That makes it harder for you to justify skipping leg day and drives you to put on your workout gear, even if you might huff and puff a bit as you do so.

Most importantly, tracking your progress allows you to definitively understand how much progress you've made. It clearly shows which of your goals you've met, to what degree you've met them, and which ones you still have to achieve. That information can be used to determine if you're on the right track with your goals. If you're progressing faster than you thought, then you might adjust your goals to make them a bit more challenging. If you're progressing more slowly than you thought, you can adjust your goals to make them more achievable and realistic for you.

To reap these benefits, you'll need to properly keep track of your progress. There are a number of ways you can do so. For instance, you can take your body measurements using a flexible tape once a week or once a month. Then, you can record the results in a notebook and see how your body changes over time. In this way, you can clearly see if you're meeting your body composition goals or not.

Another way to track your progress is to test your rep max. If you hit the gym, you likely do several movements and repeat them a number of times. These repetitions are called reps. Your rep max is the most number of reps you can comfortably do. The longer you regularly work out, the stronger your muscles will become. The stronger your muscles become, the higher your rep max will be. By testing your rep max on a biweekly or monthly basis, you can keep track of how much stronger your muscles have gotten and how far you've come. As a rule, you should do a couple of different exercises to test your rep max. These exercises must use different groups of muscles. Otherwise, you won't get a full and accurate picture of your progress.

How about your aerobic progress? One way to track this would be to take your blood pressure once a month, every month. This way, you can ensure heart health and see just how much your aerobic exercises are benefitting your heart and cardiovascular system. You can also use a fitness tracker of some sort, such as a Fitbit. These trackers can record your aerobic fitness progress, like how far and fast you're able to run or cycle. It can lay this information out in a graphic of some sort so you can take a quick snapshot of your progress. You can then go ahead and celebrate how far you've come.

Speaking of, celebrating your progress and the milestones you achieve is a must. This is because such celebrations can be additional sources of motivation. It can allow you to take pride in what you've accomplished through dedication and effort and give you something to look forward to. Now, this doesn't mean you should eat an entire cake after meeting a fitness goal, of course. It does, however, mean you can give yourself some type of reward that you know you'll enjoy. This is an especially good idea for meeting fitness goals that involve doing activities you don't particularly enjoy and would love to avoid. In such cases, the promise of a reward can make the trial you're about to go through infinitely more bearable and even, dare I say, appealing.

# Chapter 3:

# Nutrition and Diet for Optimal

# Health

In addition to working out regularly, leading a fit and healthy life in your 50s and beyond requires eating meals capable of nurturing your body. Eating a healthy, balanced diet is of the utmost importance for everyone, not just people who are in their 50s. However, for those who have hit the big 5–0, a balanced diet can be especially important because it has a myriad of benefits to offer you. In essence, a balanced diet keeps you healthy in the following ways (Crichton-Stuart, 2020):

- A balanced diet keeps your blood pressure low, your heart strong, and your cardiovascular system healthy.

- It keeps your bad cholesterol level down, further protecting your heart and cardiovascular system and reducing your risk of developing heart disease.

- It reduces your risk of developing different types of cancer.

- It improves your gut health by decreasing inflammation in the gut and increasing the number of good bacteria in your gut— yes, they exist—which do all sorts of good things for your body, like produce vitamins B and K.

- It improves your memory, thanks to the rich vitamin D, C, and E content and high omega-3 fatty acid content that healthy, whole foods come with.

- It lowers blood sugar levels, blood pressure levels, and cholesterol levels, thereby protecting against diabetes and heart disease.

- It strengthens your bones and teeth and reduces your risk of experiencing bone diseases such as osteoporosis.

# Importance of a Balanced Diet As You Age

As you can see, eating a balanced diet is very important. It becomes even more crucial as you get older, particularly once you turn 50. Maintaining a diet from this point on will have more benefits than you can count. For example, it will slow down muscle mass and bone density loss and strengthen your muscles and bones instead. If you eat the right kind of food, you'll have an easier time producing more muscle mass (Gidus, 2011).

At the same time, maintaining a healthy diet will help keep your blood sugar levels under control—a fact you might otherwise struggle with since your metabolism slows down as you age, causing there to be more glucose in your blood. This process increases your risk of diabetes, as you know, but it doesn't have to be the case. You can keep your blood sugar level under control by eating healthy foods and portioning them correctly. Hint: The portion sizes you'll have to eat to watch your blood sugar level and your weight at age 55 will be smaller than the portions you ate at 25.

A healthy diet is also important as you age because many people experience vitamin C and B deficiencies, alongside some mineral deficiencies. This process usually starts happening in a person's 50s and 60s. By eating the right kinds of varied, healthy foods, people can get ahead of these deficiencies.

A proper diet can be very beneficial for your cognitive capabilities, such as your memory, too. As you've learned, your memory and other cognitive capabilities can start declining a bit as you age. Eating certain foods can help. The nutrients in healthy, whole foods can ensure that your brain stays healthy and fit in its own way. On top of that, it can reduce your risk of experiencing Alzheimer's or dementia.

A final benefit that healthy eating might offer you is that it can boost your immune system. Your immune system, which protects you against illnesses, weakens as you age. By eating the right foods with the right nutrients, such as vitamin C, you can strengthen your immune system. You can help it protect you from illnesses and make it easier for it to fight off an illness when you do get sick at one point or another.

## Nutritional Needs Specific to Gay Men Over 55

So, what does a healthy, balanced diet mean for you, specifically? To answer this question, we first have to cover what nutrients are. Nutrients are the various substances that are found in the foods that you eat. Your body typically needs these nutrients because they help maintain its health and strength and keep things working as they should. Typically speaking, there are six types of nutrients the human body needs, no matter how many years that body has been on planet Earth (Fletcher, 2019):

- vitamins

- minerals

- fats

- protein

- carbs

- water

Vitamins can more accurately be described as micronutrients. They come in many shapes and sizes, though they're all tiny, as you might have figured from the "micro" part of "micronutrients." Different vitamins are good for different things in your body, of course, but here's an overview of their general benefits:

- strengthen the immune system

- protect against various kinds of cancer, including prostate cancer

- help your body absorb the mineral known as calcium better

- strengthen your bones and teeth

- ensure you have a healthy circulation system

- make it easier for your body to metabolize and breakdown proteins and carbs

- improve your skin health so you're glowing

- improve your brain and nervous system functioning

As for how many kinds of vitamins there are, that would be 13 in all. Some of these vitamins are fat-soluble vitamins, meaning that they dissolve in fat. Fat-soluble vitamins are vitamins A, K, E, and D. The remaining nine vitamins are water-soluble ones. These are vitamins B-12, B1, B6, B2, B5 B3, B7, B9, and C.

Then there are your minerals. Minerals are also micronutrients, and like vitamins, your body needs them. These minerals are typically grouped into two categories: major and minor vitamins. First, here are the major minerals you'll want to ensure you're consuming:

- magnesium

- calcium

- phosphorus

- potassium

- sulfur

- sodium

- chloride

These minerals help you balance out the water level inside your body, strengthen your bones, take care of them, and improve your skin, nail, and hair health. Here are the minor minerals to include in your diet:

- manganese

- zinc

- iron

- selenium

- chromium

- fluoride

- iodine

- molybdenum

- copper

Before you ask, no, this isn't a list of materials needed for a construction project. Your body needs these minor minerals because they keep you from getting cavities, strengthen your bones, help your circulatory system get oxygen across your body, improve your blood pressure, and prevent blood clotting.

Now, onto fats and carbs. For years, we've been sold the fiction that fats and carbs are our enemies. Surprise: They're not. They're key nutrients that our bodies need to function properly—though obviously in moderation. You see, fats and carbs are essential sources of energy for us. Without them, we can't muster the energy needed to go about our day. Without fats and carbs, our bodies can't function the way they're supposed to, either. Take fats, for example. Healthy fats serve a lot of functions in our bodies. They help our cells to grow properly and create new ones. They help with blood clotting, reduce our risk of developing type 2 diabetes and heart disease, and maintain normal blood sugar levels. At the same time, they support the healthy functioning of our brain, make it easier for our muscles to move, aid our body's mineral and vitamin absorption abilities, facilitate hormone production, and strengthen our immune system.

Carbs are essential for your health, too. More accurately, complex carbs are essential for your health. On the one hand, complex carbs take longer to digest and give you more energy over long periods of time. On the other hand, simple carbs are digested very quickly but only provide you with short bursts of energy. In this regard, complex carbs are like a well-maintained fire, whereas simple carbs are like lit matchsticks—they'll blow out in a moment or two (Kandola, 2019).

So, as a rule, you want to consume complex carbs more often than simple ones. By doing so, you'll provide your body with all the energy it needs throughout the day. You'll also enjoy some of the other benefits that complex carbs have to offer you, like strengthening your immune system, improving your brain functioning, improving your digestive system's functioning, and strengthening your nervous system.

Then, there's protein. Protein is a must for anyone, but especially for aging men. This is because you need protein to keep building muscle, and you need to keep building muscle if you are to get ahead of the muscle mass loss that comes with age. Protein isn't just vital for that, though. It's also essential for ensuring the health and proper development of your bones, skin, and hair and your ability to form new and healthy hormones and antibodies (Fletcher, 2019). Protein also serves as a power source for your cells and tissues, though it's only used as needed. Remember, your primary energy sources are healthy fats and complex carbs, so don't cut those out of your life!

The final nutrient you need in your life is water. By that, I don't mean that you should drink plenty of iced tea and coffee throughout the day. Yes, those do have some water content, but what we really need is pure, clear, filtered water. As human beings, we need water to survive, so much so that we can only go three days, at most, without it. We want to avoid dehydration because it has some unpleasant side effects like headaches, and a lack of water can severely impact our body's ability to function properly.

Our bodies need water for many things. It flushes out the harmful toxins that sneak their way into our bodies. It provides us with shock absorption, which comes in very handy when we experience a fall. It keeps us from becoming constipated, lubricates our joints so we can move them comfortably, and helps transport the other nutrients we consume to different parts of our bodies.

## Nutrients Gay Men Over 55 Need

Here's a question for you. There's no doubt that we all need these different nutrients to ensure our strength and keep us strong. Are there any nutrients that you specifically need as you age, though? Are there any nutrients that you should consume more or less of? If so, what foods should you eat to do so? Alright, that was more than one question, but they're valid ones to ask. So, let's take our time answering them.

To answer that first question, yes, there are specific nutrients you need to consume as you age since these will be immensely beneficial for you. You'll want to ensure the following nutrients are in your diet:

- fiber, which is a type of complex carb

- protein—shocking, I know

- calcium, which is a mineral, as you'll recall

- potassium, which is yet another mineral you need

- folate, otherwise known as vitamin B-9

- vitamin D, which you were probably expecting to see on this list

Fiber is a type of complex carb. However, unlike a lot of carbs, it's not something your body can digest. Why must you eat more of it, then?

That's because fiber helps your digestive system to function better. For example, if you're constipated, adding more fiber to your diet will help you immensely. Fiber helps with a lot of other things, too. Studies show that fiber improves physical activity and performance (Wirth, 2022). They also show that it increases your lifespan, improves your cognitive abilities, meaning your brain's ability to function, and decreases the risk that you'll experience heart disease. If you are over 51 years old, then experts recommend that you, as a man, eat 28 grams of fiber per day.

Protein is definitely among those nutrients you must consume more of as you age because it helps you build muscle and slows down or even prevents muscle mass loss. If left unchecked, muscle mass loss can severely impact your ability to go about your daily life. It can also increase your risk of experiencing some sort of heart disease or developing diabetes. The way to prevent such things is simple: work out regularly and eat more protein. Specifically, try to eat at least between 30 to 35 grams of protein every day, ideally within two hours after you're done with your workout (Shetty, 2024).

Calcium is an essential ingredient for bone and teeth health, as you saw. Meanwhile, bone density loss is a common occurrence that comes with age. To prevent it, you have to do things that strengthen your bones, which means consuming more calcium. As a man over 51 years old, "more" means at least 1,000 milligrams per day.

It's obvious why we need more calcium as we age. Why we need potassium might not be as obvious, though. After all, we grew up hearing all about how good milk and calcium are for us, not potassium. Yet, potassium is one of the most beneficial minerals we can consume for our health. This is because potassium helps with muscle contractions and improves our brains' cognitive abilities. At the same time, it decreases the risk that we'll develop conditions such as heart disease, kidney stones, and high blood pressure and the risk that we'll have a stroke. Now, most experts recommend you consume about 4,700 milligrams of potassium per day. However, everyone's body is a little different. So, asking your primary care physician how much potassium you need might be the way to go here.

How about folates? Folate is the fancy term for vitamin B-9. This vitamin is essential for your health because it improves cognitive functioning and hearing, both of which can become impaired with age. Folates can also reduce your risk of developing Alzheimer's or a similar cognitive condition and depression. For this to be the case, you have to consume about 500 milligrams of folate per day.

Last but not least, we have vitamin D. Consuming more vitamin D can help you avoid osteoporosis, otherwise known as brittle bone disease. Furthermore, it can reduce your risk of developing a heart condition and ending up with high blood pressure. It can even prevent cognitive decline as you age and keep you mentally sharp. If you're over 51, then you must consume 600 international units (IU) of vitamin D every day.

Just as there are certain nutrients you should consume more of, there are ones you should eat less of as well. Chief among these are carbs and fats. This doesn't mean you should cut these two things out of your diet. It just means that you should reduce your intake. This makes sense when you think about it: If your metabolism slows down with age, then consuming the same amounts of energy-giving food, like carbs and fats, will mean ending up with excess energy. That will result in your blood sugar level being high. It will also mean your body will store all that extra energy, which is why your waist size will start getting bigger.

If you don't want to end up with that kind of pot belly situation but want to keep fit instead, then you need to consume less carbs and fats. But what does it look like? That depends entirely on how active you are. If you're going to be working out—and I'm assuming you intend to do that, you picked up this book—then your carb intake will depend on how intense your workout is. If you're going for moderate exercise and lead a moderately active lifestyle, then your daily caloric intake should be 2,400 calories. If you're performing intense activities and leading a very active lifestyle, though, it should be 2,800 calories. This is only true if you're between the ages of 51 and 55, though. If you're between 55 and 66, though, your carb intake should be 2,400 calories for a moderately active lifestyle and 2,600 calories for an active lifestyle (*What Older Adults Should Know*, 2021).

What about healthy fats? Like carbs, there are different types of fats: monosaturated fats, polyunsaturated fats (which consist of omega-3s and omega-6s), saturated fats, and trans fats. Of these different types, saturated fats and trans fats are found in fast food and pre-packaged foods. Hence, they're unhealthy fats you want to avoid as much as possible, especially since they can raise your cholesterol levels and your risk of developing heart disease. Alternatively, polyunsaturated fats, omega-3s, and omega-6s are fats that are quite good for you (*Healthy Eating over 60*, 2020). Monounsaturated fats, which are found in nuts, seeds, olive oil, and canola oil, lower your cholesterol levels.

Polyunsaturated fats are the essential fats you need as your body can't produce them. Hence, you need to get them from the food you eat. Of these, omega-3s protect your heart from heart disease and can be found in olive oil, seafood, flaxseed, and nuts. Meanwhile, omega-6s can be found in sunflower seeds and soybean oils.

As before, how much fat you need depends on how much exercise you're getting. If you're getting a lot of exercise, especially with the intention of putting on some muscle mass, then at 55, you should consume between 55 and 99 grams of healthy fats. If you're leading a less active lifestyle and are actually trying to maintain your weight, then at 55, you should consume between 40 and 80 grams per day (*Fat Intake Calculator*, n.d.). If you want to get a little more specific than that, then you're going to have to either pay a visit to your trainer or primary care physician or take out your calculator and do some math. Factors like your height, weight, and activity level will go a long way in determining how much fat you should consume per day.

## Strategies for Maintaining a Healthy Weight and Reducing Chronic Diseases

Now that we've examined what your body needs as you age, let's translate what we've learned into more practical terms and answer the question, "What should I eat?" As a rule, you want to maintain the kind of diet that meets all these nutritional needs we've covered. That means eating some very specific foods. For instance, you know you need to eat more protein as you age, but what type of protein should you eat?

Well, you want to go for options that have high protein counts and don't have a lot of, if any, unhealthy fats in them. In the following list, you'll find the best foods that meet this description (Davidson, 2021):

- fish

- poultry

- lean meats

- eggs

- tofu

- lentils

- beans

- seeds and nuts

- dairy products

- tempeh

Next up, we have fiber. You can find plenty of that in fruits and vegetables, which have the added benefit of being rich in vitamins and minerals. You can also get lots of fiber from whole grains, lentils, beans, nuts, and seeds.

What about those specific minerals and vitamins you need as you age, like calcium and vitamin D? To start with calcium, you can consume lots of it by eating dairy products and leafy greens, with the exception of spinach, and drinking soy milk or almond milk. Meanwhile, you can find plenty of potassium in bananas, leafy greens, including spinach this time, vine fruits like tomatoes, root vegetables such as potatoes, and peas and beans (*Foods High in Potassium*, 2021).

Vitamin D is something you can get plenty of by stepping out into the sun because contact with the sun starts a kind of chemical process within our bodies that makes them produce this vitamin. However, you can also get vitamin D from egg yolks, fatty fish, and mushrooms. You can take a supplement for it, too (Davidson, 2021).

Incorporating these foods into your regular diet is a good idea to maintain your health and well-being. It's also a sound strategy for maintaining a healthy weight and protecting yourself against any chronic diseases, such as diabetes. Another sound strategy for this is to work out regularly, as we've already covered. Another way to do this is to make sure you get enough sleep and rest throughout the day or, rather, at night. If you're between 18 and 61 years old, you need to get at least seven hours of sleep per night. You might think sleep is unrelated to your weight and health, but you'd be wrong. Getting enough sleep is something that actually improves the pace and functioning of your metabolism, as well as of your whole body. It maximizes your ability to burn through the calories you consume, ensuring you don't end up with any unwanted excess to store. Studies show that proper sleep also reduces your risk of developing chronic conditions such as diabetes, high blood pressure, heart conditions, and the probability that you'll have a stroke (*About Sleep*, 2024). Proper sleep even strengthens your immune system, making sure that you get sick less often and are able to recover from illnesses more quickly.

A final strategy you can adopt to maintain a healthy weight and keep chronic conditions away is to learn to manage your stress levels. One reason for this is that stress can interfere with the quality and duration of your sleep, preventing you from getting enough of it (*Coping with Stress*, 2023). Another is that it can cause chronic physical ailments like regular headaches and digestive issues. Still, another is that it can worsen any chronic conditions you already have by putting an extra toll on your body and lowering the effectiveness of your cardiovascular system. By managing your stress, you can ensure such things don't happen. You can ensure you remain calm and collected throughout the day. How to manage your stress will be the subject of another chapter entirely. However, you might be interested to know that working out regularly actually helps lower stress levels and prevents stress from becoming chronic, which is yet another reason why you want to keep exercising.

Chapter 4:

# Building Strength and Muscle

# Mass

By now, you know how important it is for us to work out as we age, but we haven't yet discussed what exercises we should be doing. I don't mean which activities—like running, push-ups, or jumping jacks—we should do. Instead, I'm referring to the different *types* of exercises we should be incorporating into our workout schedule. If you're wondering what those different types are, exercises can generally be divided into three categories: strength training, cardio, and flexibility and mobility exercises. To start, let's take a look at what strength training is and why we even need to do it.

## The Benefits of Strength Training

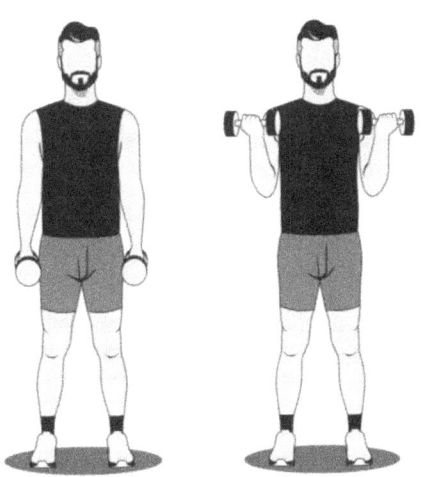

Strength or resistance training is the catch-all term for all exercises involving using weights or the weight of your own body—which is preferable to having the weight of the world on your shoulders—to train your muscles. These exercises really make your muscles burn, and you have to work different groups of muscles in various sets.

Now, they make it look a little tedious, but strength training exercises are a must, especially once you hit 50. There are several reasons why, and the most obvious is that strength training builds muscle. Doing strength training for just 20 minutes per week is enough for people between the ages of 50 and 90 to rebuild their muscles; at least, that's what study after study has found. But that's not all. Studies have also discovered that strength training can speed up your metabolism while allowing your muscles to recover more quickly after workout sessions (*13 Benefits of Strength Training for People Older than 50*, n.d.). At the same time, it can keep your body from holding onto the excess energy you consume as fat. In other words, strength training can keep you from getting, well, fat.

Speaking of fat, you now know that you need to consume a certain amount of fats as part of your diet. As a result, your blood has a certain fat content. Only this fat content is officially known as your *lipid content*, so why not have two different names for the same thing? You want your blood lipid content to be below a certain level. Otherwise, you end up with cholesterol issues and heart problems. Fortunately, strength training helps with this process. It keeps your bad cholesterol level, known as LDL cholesterol, low and your good cholesterol level, known as HDL cholesterol, high.

Strength training has some additional benefits for your heart. For example, it strengthens your heart muscles and your cardiovascular system while strengthening your muscles and bones. As a result of this process, your risk of developing some sort of heart disease goes down. At the same time, your ability to recover from heart disease, in the event that you do experience one, improves. On top of that, strength training reduces your chances of developing type 2 diabetes. Scientists have observed that people who are more muscular and fit end up being more sensitive to insulin and have better blood sugar levels, you see. They also have an easier time managing pain and, in fact, experience pain and discomfort much less often. Suppose that you deal with lower back pain. If so, strengthening your back muscles through resistance training will help. It'll reduce the pain or discomfort you feel and make it so you live more comfortably.

Speaking of muscles, resistance training slows down the rate at which your muscle cells age! It even makes you more resistant to certain kinds of cancer while making you a lot more mobile and independent. After all, stronger muscles mean greater ability to do the things you want to do, when you want to do them, without having to rely on others to help you physically.

## Safe and Effective Exercises for Building Strength

With all that information out of the way, the obvious question to ask is, "How?" How are you supposed to build strength and muscle? More specifically, what strength training exercises should you do to build muscle?

While there are an array of different strength exercises you can try and adopt to increase your strength and mobility, some tend to be better, or at least more ideal, than others. Before we dive into those exercises, though, let's first cover what you need to do to practice those exercises safely.

I'm sure you've heard of the saying "No pain, no gain" before. Macho-sounding though it may be, it is a somewhat accurate saying. It applies to strength training, where you want to feel your muscles burn. What you don't want is to feel actual pain in any way. If you do, stop whatever you're doing immediately instead of pushing through. Think of pain as a warning sign—your body is telling you something is wrong. Your body is telling you to stop so that things don't get worse. Suppose that you're lifting some weights when suddenly you feel a sharp pain zip through your elbow. This is joint pain, and it might mean several things. For example, it might be a sign that you sprained something. It might alternatively indicate some other injury or just convey that you've put too much strain on yourself. Whatever that pain means, it's a clear sign that you should stop, put away the dumbbells, and rest. If you keep going, you might end up with a really bad injury.

If you want to make sure you're safe when training, one thing to remember is to warm up before each exercise and start slow. Warming up is important because it gradually increases the blood and, therefore, oxygen flow to your muscles. So, it gradually gets your muscles to a state where they can handle the workout you're about to undertake. Thus, it reduces the risk that you'll injure yourself in some way.

Starting your workout sessions slowly is just as important as warming up for them. As a rule, you don't want to get started with your most difficult exercises, but you should do the most reps. Starting things out with intense exercises would be courting injury, especially if you're new to working out. Instead, you want to start slowly, focusing on getting each movement and exercise right. Getting things right is crucial because it'll ensure you don't make mistakes that could potentially lead to injury. Working out in front of a mirror can be very helpful. It can ensure you get things like your posture and stance right and fix any mistakes you spot, that is, if you don't get swept away by the fine-looking gentleman staring back at you.

Before you work, you should ensure that you're in as safe an environment as you can be. That means a place free of clutter that you might stumble over. It also means working out on a firm surface. So, if you're thinking of exercising on that rug that always slips around, that's probably a bad idea. Another bad idea is not wearing sneakers, as they have soles that will grip the ground properly and ensure your feet have the arch support they need. Speaking of clothing, it's essential that you don't wear clothing that is too loose, too. Tighter-fitting clothing will ensure your sleeves and hems can't get caught on something, causing you to trip and fall.

As for which exercises you should adopt, well, you can never go wrong with the ones outlined below.

### Squats

Squats are a great exercise to get into because they work out your back, leg, glute—yes, I mean your butt—and thigh muscles. To start, you want to stand with your feet just a little more than hip-length apart. Then, stand up straight, which means pushing your chest out just a bit and your shoulders back without flaring your ribcage. As you take a breath, you want to squeeze your abdominal muscles and keep your pelvis and spine stable. Hinge at your hips and slowly start bending at the knees. As you do so, lower your booty, for lack of a better word, toward the ground. Pretend there's something behind you you'd like to sit down on. As you go down, make sure your spine remains straight, don't arch backward, and don't round your shoulders (Dawn Neumann, 2016).

To answer the age-old question, "How low can you go?" you want to keep going for so long as you can comfortably sink down. You've gone too far if you feel any discomfort beyond some muscle burn. If you have any knee problems, you don't want to sink lower than 90 degrees. Hence, you want to keep your thighs and your bum parallel to the ground. Now, you might struggle a bit with your balance as you pop a squat, and that's okay. Raising your arms in front of you, at chest level, should help with this. As you sink down, your weight should be on your heels and mid-foot.

Once you've gone as low as you can go, it'll be time to come back up. To do so, you will need to press on your heels. This movement will work your glutes and hamstrings as you revert back to your original standing position. Once you're there, you can sink back down and do about 10 to 15 reps of this move.

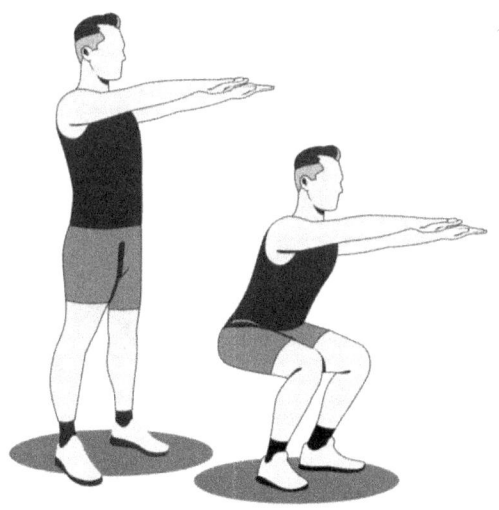

## *Dumbbell Overhead Press*

The dumbbell overhead press is a great upper-body exercise, but it's especially good for your triceps and shoulder muscles. So, it's perfect for your ability to lift and reach for things and for your posture (Rogers, 2022). Grab a dumbbell in each hand to start. Your thumbs should be on the inside of the dumbbells, and your knuckles should be facing up. This positioning is called an overhand grip, and as you maintain this grip, you want to hold your dumbbells over your shoulders and keep your elbows tucked in. If you got that posture right, stand up straight with your feet shoulder-length apart. Then, take a deep breath and exhale as you slowly raise the dumbbells overhead. Once you reach the peak, pause for a second. Inhale again as you lower the dumbbells to the previous position.

If you'd like, you can also perform this exercise while sitting. This position might be the ideal option for you if you're new to working out or have any back injuries or problems you're dealing with. For this version of the exercise, you'll need to sit on a firm surface, such as a chair or a bench. By doing so, you'll stabilize your back. Then, you'll repeat the exact same arm movements described above.

Whichever version of the exercise you do, try to avoid locking your elbows when you reach the peak. Instead, keep them slightly loose. Refrain from hunching your shoulders and arching your back. Most importantly, try to go slow. The point of this exercise isn't speed. It's getting it right during the 10 to 15 reps you do.

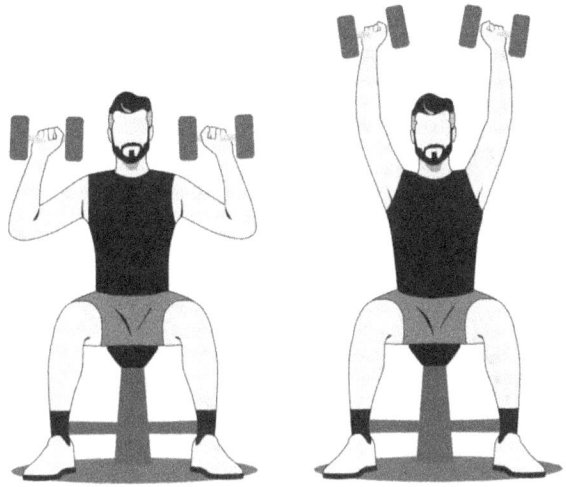

## Bench Press

A bench press is another great upper body exercise to try. It works the triceps, deltoids, chest muscles, and front muscles in general. You can do this movement with a barbell or dumbbells, but if you're new to this movement, I'd recommend using dumbbells (Williams, 2018).

To start, lie down on your back, on a bench with your feet planted firmly on the ground, not the bench. This placement ensures you'll be able to press down on your heels while you lift—more on that in a bit. Once you lie down, you can grab your dumbbells like you gripped them when you were doing overhead presses. Hold them directly over your shoulders, with your elbows at a 45-degree angle, lower than your shoulders. You never want your elbows to be parallel to your shoulders, so watch out for that. As you raise the dumbbells toward the ceiling, you're going to want to press your shoulders down onto the bench and turn the pits of your elbows toward your head. This technique will protect your shoulders from any undue stress and pain.

Again, as you lift the dumbbells, you'll want to keep your forearms perpendicular to the ground. While you lower and raise them, you want to keep the distance between the dumbbells more or less the same, never getting closer or drifting too far apart. As you lift, you should exhale and press down on your heels while tightening your abdominal muscles and keeping your shoulders back. As you lower the dumbbells to your starting position, you should inhale and go slowly. You don't want your arms to suddenly drop to the point you started at. When you are back at your starting position, you want to do six to eight reps, remembering to breathe the whole time.

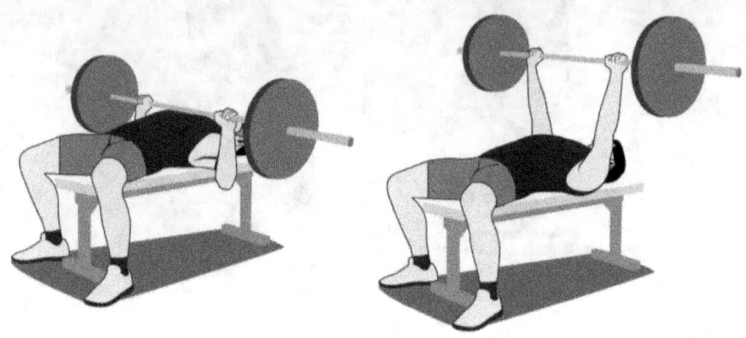

### Deadlift

A final strength training exercise to try is the deadlift, which is excellent for your glutes, back muscles, and hamstrings. Obviously, you're going to need a bar—not the kind where you can order a cocktail—to be able to perform this move. Start by walking up the bar and stop mid-foot. Your shins shouldn't be touching the bar yet, but your heels should be hip-length apart, with your toes pointing slightly out at about a 15-degree angle.

Next, you want to bend down and grab the bar, placing your hands shoulder-length apart. Once you're in that position, you can bend your knees until your shins are, at last, touching the bar. Once they do, you should take care not to let the bar move away from your mid-foot. If it does, you'll have to start from square one.

Now, if you get the position correctly, you can move on to the next step: raise your chest and straighten your back without moving yet. Then, when you're ready, you can take a deep breath and hold it. Holding your breath, you'll need to stand up with the weight, keeping it touching your legs. Once you're up, you'll want to lock your knees and hips, but refrain from shrugging or leaning back. To lower the weight, you'll need to unlock your knees and hips first. With that out of the way, you can lower the bar while keeping your knees mostly straight. You can bend your knees once the bar reaches a little below them and place it on the floor. It should land right over your mid-foot.

Once you've placed the bar on the ground, do not move. Instead, keep your hands on the bar for your next rep but do take a few seconds to breathe before you start again. Then, take a deep breath and repeat the whole movement again, doing six to eight reps like that.

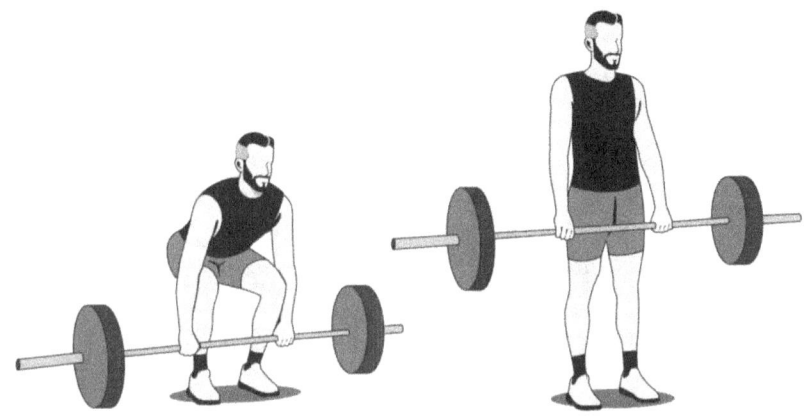

## *Workouts for Individual Fitness Levels*

Regardless of which strength of training exercises you adopt, it's important that you adopt a workout schedule that fits your fitness level. What exactly does that mean? Well, suppose that you are a beginner when it comes to strength training. If so, you're going to have to give yourself some time to get used to your workouts as you do them. This will mean you have to follow the below steps (Waehner, 2022):

- **Start slow:** Start slowly and with less heavy weights, at least for your initial training sessions. Choose full-body exercises like squats over ones that work only one part of your body. This way, you'll get to improve your overall strength more quickly.

- **Take plenty of breaks:** Give yourself some extra recovery days in your initial few weeks to give your muscles all the time they need to rest, knit themselves back together, and get stronger. Learn to listen to your body so that you can tell the difference between regular post-workout soreness and pain from overdoing it.

- **Alternate strength training days:** Do not do strength training every single day. Instead, alternate strength training days with cardio days. By following this schedule, you'll give different muscle groups the time they need to rest without losing out on valuable workout times, and you'll reap the benefits of strength training and cardio simultaneously.

If you're at more of an intermediate level when it comes to strength training, there are different things you'll have to watch out for when designing a fitness program that works for you. The rules you need to follow might look a little something like these examples:

- **Try interval training:** Try interval training once or twice a week. Interval training is a type of exercise routine where you do really high-intensity exercises one after the other, then take breaks to calm your heartbeat. This will incorporate a little cardio into your strength training and help you develop your muscles more quickly.

- **Do cardio and strength training on the same day:** Speaking of cardio and strength training, since you're now at the intermediate level, you can do both on the same day. Start by doing your strength training exercises first. Do them for about 10 to 15 minutes. Then, use the remainder of your time to do your cardio exercises. This strategy ensures you get the 150 minutes of total workout you need per week, and make sure that you do strength training for 30 to 60 minutes per week, too. Moreover, since you are at the intermediate level now, coupling your cardio and strength training exercises like this won't be too tiring for you. In fact, once you witness how much resilience and strength you've gained, you might even find yourself enjoying it.

- **Split your strength training:** Now that you've increased your overall strength, you can focus on specific parts of your body more. A great strategy is to devote some time to upper-body strength and lower-body strength, respectively. This strategy is called splitting your training, and it can help you become much stronger more quickly. Don't skip leg day, though, unless you want to look like Gru from *Despicable Me*.

What if you're at a more advanced level? If so, that obviously means you can handle more intense activities and exercises. Here's what you'll have to watch for:

- **Mix up your workout routines:** Have you ever had a song you love that you played over and over again, only to become absolutely sick of it? If so, you know how dangerous monotony and repetition can be. They can kill even the most entertaining of things. So, it stands to reason that they can kill your enthusiasm to work out as well. However, you can avoid this occurrence by mixing up your workout routines regularly. Keep things as fresh and novel as possible. That doesn't mean you don't have to go to moves and sets, of course. It just means mixing up when you do them and not letting yourself hesitate to try new things.

- **Don't forget to rest:** While working out is important, you cannot forget that rest days are equally important because they're when your muscles repair themselves and make themselves stronger. So, make absolutely sure you give yourself the rest days you need and deserve.

- **Up your cardio, not just your strength training:** One thing you don't want to do is make your strength training more intense while keeping your cardio exercises the same. This mistake will actually hinder your progress. It will keep you from increasing your conditioning alongside your strength, which will, in turn, make it impossible for you to practice some of the more intense resistance training exercises out there—a fact that can prove immensely frustrating for you.

## Strength Training Strategies for a Healthy Weight and Managing Chronic Diseases

One of the greatest benefits of strength training is that it helps you maintain a healthy weight and manage chronic diseases. Strength training helps in these areas because of four key reasons (Godman, 2022):

1. It lowers your blood sugar level because your muscles play a part in your body's ability to store muscles. Making your muscles stronger means they will be better able to store sugars, which automatically lowers your blood sugar level.

2. It lowers your blood pressure. Having stronger muscles means having more blood vessels flow through those muscle fibers, which takes a significant amount of pressure off of your cardiovascular system.

3. It helps you burn more calories because your muscles use calories 24 hours a day. Having more muscles translates to having more components to burn more energy calories.

4. It reduces inflammation across the body. The more muscles you develop, the fewer fat cells you end up with, meaning that you end up with fewer cells that actually worsen inflammation in your body.

So, what do these areas have to do with your weight and chronic diseases? Well, high blood sugar, high blood pressure, an excess of calories, and inflammation across the body typically lead to weight problems and chronic diseases of all sorts. High blood pressure, for example, often translates to chronic heart disease. High blood sugar can lead to chronic issues like diabetes and insulin resistance, as can inflammation. Inflammation can lead to other chronic diseases, too, like rheumatoid arthritis, heart disease, and asthma, to give a few examples. Meanwhile, an excess of calories often leads to excess weight and sometimes even obesity.

Doing strength training for just 30 to 60 minutes per week, however, can prevent all this from happening. It can help you maintain a healthy weight and reduce your risk of developing chronic diseases. However, getting into strength training can be a little tough, especially if you're not used to it. This reason is why you should start small and slow, meaning you shouldn't go with the heaviest weights but instead work your way up to them. You shouldn't go with the lightest ones either. As a rule, if you want to build muscle, then you must start with weights that are equal to or greater than 60% of your rep max (Edwards, 2022). Start by testing your rep max with different weights. Once you've settled on a weight, keep practicing with it, doing up to eight repetitions and between one to three sets overall. If you've chosen the right weights, then you should get to the point where you can't lift anymore with those weights after that many reps. If, after some practice, you reach a point where you can keep going after that many reps, congratulations! You're ready to move onto even heavier weights!

One thing you want to focus on as you're doing your various strength training exercises is your form. All those reps and sets will mean little if you get your stance and form wrong. At best, you'll end up working the wrong muscle groups or making your workout less effective. At worst, you'll end up injuring yourself. So, be sure to pay close attention to your form as you work, and don't rush through your movements. Similarly, try to adopt compound movements, meaning exercises that work for different muscle groups at the same time as much as possible. Squats and bench presses are great examples of such moves. These will offer you greater benefits than exercise focusing on single muscle groups ever can (Carter, 2022).

A final strategy you must adopt when strength training is to be sure to always warm up and cool down. Warm-ups prepare your muscles for the workout they're about to do, thereby reducing your chance of injuring yourself and making the exercises you're about to do just a bit easier for you. Cool-downs are equally important for settling your heart rate and breathing following an intense strength training regimen. These will allow you to turn off workout mode and get back to your daily life. They will also make it easier for your body, especially your worn and torn muscles, to go into repair and recovery mode.

# Chapter 5:

# Cardiovascular Health and

# Endurance

Cardiovascular exercises—otherwise known simply as cardio or aerobic exercises—should be included in *everyone's* routine. However, they're especially important as you get older. If you're like me and hate running, that's not the best news. Fortunately, cardio doesn't just mean running. This category of exercises includes all different types, and some of them can be quite fun. The trick is to find activities that you enjoy and can fit into your lifestyle. Before you get there, though, let's cover what cardio exercises are.

Cardio exercises get your heart beating fast. When this happens, your body starts pumping a great deal of oxygen throughout your body. Similarly, it starts burning a lot of calories and fat. Everyone can do cardio, but everyone's capacity for cardio is a little different. For example, your genetics wield a 20–40% influence over your cardiovascular capabilities (Waehner, 2019). Your age plays an important role in this process, too, since your cardiovascular capabilities decrease as you age. That doesn't mean that getting older will keep you from doing cardio; instead, it just means it may impact the kind of cardio exercises you can do and how intense they should be. But wait—why should you care? Why should you even do cardio, especially if you're already doing strength training?

# Why Cardio Is Important

Cardio exercises are important for several reasons. For starters, they burn a lot of fat and calories. As a result, they keep you from gaining unnecessary weight and help you to keep fit. Doing cardio regularly actually helps you to sleep, too. It improves both the quality of your sleep and makes it easier for you to fall asleep, which is excellent news for those of us who have a tendency to toss and turn in bed.

Cardio workouts also improve your lung health and lung capacity, meaning the amount of air you can hold in your lungs. It increases your bone density, which is good news considering the bone density loss that comes with age. It lowers stress, too, making it infinitely more manageable and keeping you from developing chronic stress issues. Surprisingly enough, cardio has some additional mental health benefits, like lowering your anxiety and depression and helping you to feel better and more confident overall. On the more physical side of things, it improves your heart health and makes your heart and cardiovascular system stronger while reducing your blood pressure, cholesterol, and blood sugar, keeping chronic diseases at bay in the process (Waehner, 2022).

One unexpected benefit of cardio is that it improves your sex life. That fact makes sense when you think about it, especially considering what a breathless activity sex can be. However, its benefits for your sex life go beyond that. You see, doing regular cardio improves your body's ability to become aroused, and it can even help with sexual dysfunction, especially the type that's caused by certain types of medication (Brown, 2023).

Cardio has some benefits that are specific to you in your current age, too. You see, as we age, our hearts start losing some of their ability to pump blood. By the time you're 40, you lose 5% to 10% of your blood flow capacity (Ratini, 2024). By the time you're 50, you lose even more than that. Doing cardio regularly reverses that process. Hence, it keeps your heart healthy, strong, and, dare I say, even young. As an extension of that, cardio actually extends your life because it keeps both your heart and your body healthy in general. It does so by speeding up your metabolism, making it harder for you to gain weight, and keeping all your organs and systems working better and more quickly, including your brain. Cardio ends up supplying more oxygen to your brain, which helps keep it in tip-top shape. That improves your cognitive abilities, such as your memory and ability to think.

Having said that, you must approach cardio with some caution once you've hit 50. Injuries happen more easily as you age, and cardio is the kind of exercise where you might suffer an accident easily. If you've gone for a jog, for example, you might trip and fall. Hence, you should always be very aware of your surroundings while you're doing cardio. You should also talk to your doctor before drawing up an aerobic exercise program for yourself, especially if you have a previous injury or a previous health condition. Even without such things, you must immediately stop working out if you feel yourself getting dizzy, experiencing shortness of breath, feeling a sharp pain in your chest, getting sores that aren't healing, or experiencing swelling of the joints. You should similarly stop working out if you get a hernia for obvious reasons.

## *Different Types of Cardio for Gay Men Over 55*

Obviously, you should always do cardio, no matter what your age, but cardio becomes especially important as you age. That begs the question: What kind of cardio exercises should you do? Are there any ones you should avoid once you hit 55? Are there ones you should especially do?

So, here's something you might not have known about cardio: There are actually two types. The first type is high-impact cardio. The second type is low-impact cardio. High-impact cardio is an aerobic exercise that has a lot of impact on your joints and feet. Running and jumping, for example, are high-impact cardiovascular exercises. Therefore, they're among those cardio exercises you want to avoid as you age. Low-impact cardio exercises do the exact opposite. They put very little strain and have very little impact on your joints like your knees. Hence, they're the kind of cardio you want to be doing.

So, high-impact aerobic exercises are among those moves that you should typically avoid. These moves include anything from running to running stairs and jumping. Tennis is also a high-impact sport, but it's among the more permissible options available to you, at least at 55. At 75, however, it might not be the best sport for you to engage in.

By now, you're probably wondering this question: *What cardio should I do?* First and foremost, you should make a point of walking. By that, I don't mean you should stroll for two hours to cover a distance you could walk in 10 minutes. No, I mean brisk walking for at least 30 minutes a day. Now, you might scoff at this suggestion. After all, it's only walking, right? What good is that going to do? Plenty! For starters, brisk walking, the kind that gets you slightly winded, is great for burning and therefore decreasing body fat. It's known to improve your balance, which makes it harder for you to experience a fall or injury, and strengthen your bones and muscles. It even lessens your risk of having a stroke or suffering heart disease while increasing your endurance and heart health (Mellardo, 2022).

There's also an additional mental health benefit to walking: It can reduce your stress level significantly and make it easier for you to manage your emotions. This is especially true for walking in nature or at least somewhere outside, like a park. Studies show that being out in or around nature for just 10 minutes improves mental health a lot. It lowers stress levels and blood pressure, soothes brain activity, thereby preventing overthinking, improves cognitive functioning, meaning your ability to think and do things, and even improves the quality and duration of your sleep (Jimenez, 2021).

What if you don't like walking, though? What if you find it boring despite all the people-watching opportunities it provides you with? If that's the case, you might try jogging or hiking a chance. Both activities will get your heart rate up. If you're jogging at a slow pace, then a 45-minute journey should serve your purposes very well. If, however, you're going at a more brisk pace, lapping at the heels of running, then sticking to a 20-minute jog will be a good idea (Luff, 2022).

If being bipedal still isn't your thing, why not try swimming? Swimming is a great full-body, low-impact cardio exercise to try. It's perfect for any age but particularly well suited for you in your 50s. For one, it's very easy on your joints and is often recommended to anyone who's dealing with chronic conditions like rheumatism or arthritis. It's known to lower blood pressure and improve heart health. Studies have found that swimming is particularly beneficial for your brain. These studies have shown that men over 50 years of age have better memories, cognitive functioning, and greater mental clarity when they swim regularly (*Discover 7 Surprising Health Benefits of Swimming over 50*, 2023).

Then there's how swimming impacts your lung capacity. All cardio exercises improve your lung capacity, but this goes double for swimming. After all, it does require that you hold your breath for a bit. Swimming is so good at improving lung capacity that it can alleviate the symptoms of asthma, along with any other respiratory issues you may have.

Since we're on the topic of water-related activities, one exercise you might try is water aerobics. Yes, I know, it's an old cliche—one we've seen in plenty of movies and TV shows—but cliches are cliches for a reason. Water aerobics are popular among the 50s and over group for good reason. Globally, as of 2018, 10.52 million people regularly practiced water aerobics (*Aquatic Exercise: Number of Participants*, 2019). This is partly because being in water means actively working against resistance to move. Hence, it's something that increases your muscle and bone strength. At the same time, the movements that go along with water aerobics cause your heart rate to pick up. So, they prove to be a good cardiovascular workout, except without putting any strain on your joints (Walters, 2024).

Another low-impact, full-body cardio exercise you can try is cycling either outdoors on an actual bike or indoors on a stationary bike. But how hard should you ride? To be clear, you don't want to be left completely out of breath and drenched in sweat by the time you're done. Instead, you want to ride at an intensity where your mouth gapes slightly open, and you're puffing and panting a bit. However, you should still be able to close your mouth and breathe in and out through your nose. If you can't do that, you're pushing it and may want to scale it down some. If you're not even a little out of breath, you may want to pick a fast-paced song on your playlist—I'd recommend Madonna's *Vogue*—and pick up a little speed, trying to keep pace with it (Brett, 2023).

If you want to try your hand at something that's a little more unique and will offer the added benefit of improving your balance and flexibility alongside your cardiovascular endurance, then tai chi may be just for you. Tai chi is a perfect aerobic exercise for those over 50. Not only does it reduce blood pressure and improve your brain health and heart health, but it actually can ease pain—particularly joint pain—and prevent falls.

Tai chi is an ancient, traditional Chinese practice that combines a series of artistic-looking, slow movements with controlled breathing and various postures. Some people consider tai chi to be a form of moving meditation, which means that it is immensely relaxing and makes your heart beat faster. That may sound like a contradiction to some, but it's not. After all, it's not stress that's making your heart beat faster—it's just some movement (Crouch, 2024).

It wouldn't be appropriate to introduce tai chi as an activity you can try but fail to mention dance. There are many reasons why you should get into dance if you can. For one, dancing increases your lung capacity, muscular strength, and bone density. In addition, it increases your spatial awareness and improves your balance. This naturally reduces your risk of falling, tripping over something, knocking something over, or otherwise injuring yourself. Dancing improves the way you can carry your weight and hold your posture, too. It increases your flexibility and is known to improve osteoporosis if you have it. On top of all that, dancing is a very social activity, and there are many different kinds of dance you can try. For example, you can try ballroom dancing or some other couples' dance with your partner and rekindle your romance in the process. Alternatively, you can go to rock and roll (as if you need it) or Zumba calls with friends. Or, you can go to such classes alone and meet new people. Dancing can be a very social activity that's good for your mental health and relationships (*10 Reasons Why Dancing after 50 Is Great*, 2021).

## Tips for Improving Stamina and Endurance

Here's the thing about cardio: When you first start your workout routine, you're going to get tired quickly and easily. It's important that you don't get disheartened because this outcome is perfectly normal and to be expected. After all, you haven't developed your stamina and endurance levels yet. Think of your stamina and cardiovascular endurance as a muscle. Just as you can't walk into the gym and expect to lift the heaviest of weights without any prior strength training, you can't expect to be able to swim or cycle or do whatever it is you're doing non-stop for an hour. However, you will be able to do that eventually. You'll just have to keep developing your strength and endurance for it.

The secret is simple: Keep doing cardio regularly. Say that you've decided to try cycling. Cycle a few times a day, every day. Start slow and increase the duration and intensity of your cycling sessions bit by bit. After a few weeks have gone by, you'll notice that you can cycle continuously for longer and go faster without getting as winded. That's a sure sign your stamina and endurance are improving.

As a rule, you should do at least 20 minutes of cardio for this to be the case. But is there anything else you can do besides regularly working out to further improve your stamina and cardiovascular endurance? Of course, there are! One of these things is to drink more water. Yeah, I'm not kidding. You see, water isn't just good for keeping us alive. Water is essential for the functioning of our metabolism. The more you drink, the better and faster it can work. The better and faster your metabolism works, the more energy you end up with. Studies show that just drinking 500 ml of water per day—the equivalent of about one glass of water per hour—increases your metabolic rate by as much as 30% (*5 Tips for Improving Physical Stamina in Your 50s*, 2022). That's 30% more energy for you to use however you'd like.

Taking vitamins regularly can also help you improve your stamina and endurance. This improvement occurs because vitamins and other supplements help your metabolism and various bodily systems work better, as you saw before. They make you feel more energized, too. That said, you should always consult your physician before taking any kind of vitamin or supplement. That way, you can ensure you're taking the supplements you need in the correct dosages.

A final measure you can take to improve your endurance and stamina is to eat more frequently but in smaller portions. When we eat three large meals a day, our blood sugar levels rise pretty high. We also end up with a situation where those blood sugar levels fluctuate quite a bit, which can steal from our energy levels a ton. In other words, this type of fluctuation can leave us drained, tired, hungry, and therefore cranky or "hangry," if you will. Eating smaller portions more frequently, say six times a day or so, can fix this problem. It can keep our blood sugar levels pretty stable, and we feel more energized and ready to go all throughout the day as a result. It can also make it easier for us to maintain a healthy weight by avoiding the perils of overeating and watching our body composition, which is the subject matter of our next chapter.

# Chapter 6:

# Weight Management and Body

# Composition

Let's be honest: Growing old sucks a bit. You look in the mirror, and while you do see a strapping man before you, that man is no longer young. He has salt and pepper hair, or perhaps he's losing some of it. He has more crow's feet lining his eyes and wrinkles around his face. Liver spots have popped over his hands like daisies, and certain parts are... looking a little more saggy than they used to. Taking in and accepting these changes can be hard, especially if you used to look like a young Marlon Brando. However, it doesn't mean you're no longer good-looking. It doesn't mean you can no longer pass as striking or fabulous or whatever flattering adjective you like going by. It just means you're going to have to put in a little more work. More specifically, you're going to have to put in some work to be healthier because, let's face it, the healthier you are, the better-looking you will be. This process will require working out regularly and eating well. Most importantly, it will require managing your weight and body composition.

## Strategies for Weight Loss and Healthy Weight Management

As you may recall from earlier chapters, your body composition is the percentage of fat, muscle, and bone in your body. It's essentially a measurement you use to determine if you're at a healthy weight or not. Now, determining your body composition isn't something you can do for yourself unless you actually are a doctor who knows how. You'll need to take a trip to your physician, who'll use one of five methods to determine this factor (Wheeler, 2023):

- **Skin calipers** measure your skinfold thickness, where fat is typically stored in the body.

- A **body prod** is a machine that measures the amount of air your body displaces.

- **Underwater weighing**, for which you'll be submerged in the water because fat floats, allowing it to be weighed using some special equipment.

- **Bioelectrical impedance** is a technique that isn't as painful as it sounds. It sends electrical currents through your body and then measures their travel speed to measure your body's fat content.

- A **dual X-ray absorptiometry (DEXA) scan** sends low-level X-rays through your body to find just how much fat, muscle, and bone is in there.

As a 55-year-old gay man, you want your body composition readings to be within the following ranges (Abbate, 2019):

- Fat: 11–22%

- Muscle: 73–82%

- Bone density: 3–5%

You also want your total water percentage to be between 50–65%.

Now, if your figures are below these percentages, then you want to work to improve them. That may mean doing more strength training if your muscle and bone density percentages are low and eating more, though in a healthy way, to increase your fat content. Remember, your body needs some fat to function properly. Of course, the keyword there is "some." Too much fat disrupts your bodily functions and causes all sorts of problems, like high cholesterol and an increased risk of heart disease, as you saw. So, if your percentages are too high, you want to work—that is to say, workout—to bring them down.

Let's move on to the obvious question: How do you lose weight or maintain a healthy weight at 55? There are numerous things you can do, and most of them are related to your diet and workout routine. To start with the diet-related strategies, you can eat more fruits and vegetables, generally speaking. Studies have shown that people who eat more fruits and vegetables tend to lose more weight than those who don't, even if both groups eat healthily. This goes double for anyone who eats more cauliflowers, pears, apples, berries, and soy (Bertoia et al., 2015).

Another technique you can adopt is to eat more beans. Beans are a fantastic source of protein, and they're very rich in fiber. Their nutrient content feeds the good bacteria in your gut and makes them stronger. As a result, your metabolism picks up speed. People who eat more beans regularly lose more weight more quickly, at least according to one study (Stewart et al., 2024).

Losing and managing weight isn't just about what you eat, though. It also has a lot to do with how quickly or slowly you eat. If you eat quickly, then you usually end up consuming larger portions and more calories. If you eat slowly, you get full after consuming smaller portions and fewer calories. A great way to ensure you eat slowly is to really focus on what you eat. Try not to multitask while you eat or eat on the go. Instead, concentrate on every morsel, chew slowly and thoroughly, and try to enjoy the taste of your food as much as possible. This technique will slow the eating process down for you, and you'll end up consuming less.

Another thing that may help you to eat less is to track your food. Most of us don't realize just how much food we're eating. We end up losing track of the portions we consume and eat more than we think or mean to. Keeping track of what we eat and our portions will help. It will keep those quantities at the forefront of our minds and make clear just how many calories we're taking in. This information will allow us to make more conscious and deliberate decisions concerning both what we eat and how much of it we consume.

One of the best things you can do for your health and weight is to cut out sugary drinks from your life. Sugary drinks may not seem like a big deal, but a single can of Coke or Pepsi has 150 calories in it. They're also packed with all sorts of really harmful chemicals. Despite how many calories they contain, they do nothing to sate your hunger and make their way through your body very quickly. That last one means that they raise your blood sugar really quickly and cause it to drop just as fast. Studies have found that people who quit drinking sugary drinks, particularly things like soda, gain less weight in general and are quicker to lose weight when they try (Zheng et al., 2015).

If you really want to lose weight or maintain a healthy weight, one strategy you might want to try is intermittent fasting. Intermittent fasting requires not eating for a certain time period throughout the day (Easter, 2019). That period might be anything from eight to twelve hours. This eating style is healthy and often recommended because it triggers your body's fat-burning capabilities and improves your blood sugar levels. Hence, it may be worth a try.

Remember how we said you may want to eat six small meals per day rather than three large ones? Well, this kind of diet can certainly help you lose weight or keep to a healthy one. However, you don't have to always eat full "meals" all six times when you adopt this habit. Instead, you can just incorporate snacks into your diet, albeit healthy ones. As it happens, certain snacks are more supportive of your weight management efforts than others. Chief among them are nuts. Studies have found that adult men who regularly snack on nuts gain weight more slowly and gradually than others (Liu et al., 2019). They end up having a lower risk of developing obesity, too. Of course, this fact doesn't apply if you're eating buckets and buckets of nuts. A handful or so should suffice, at least for snack time.

Another point you may remember from earlier chapters is that carbs need to be a part of your diet if you want to be healthy and strong. However, certain carbs are better than others. It's complex carbs you need to make part of your diet rather than simple ones. This is especially true of whole grains, which, as it turns out, help you burn more calories than other types of carbs! Whole grains include foods such as quinoa, oats, and barley. They're very rich in fiber and great for your digestive system as a result. They help you to lose more weight because they get you to expel more fat when you go to the toilet. Yes, I mean in the form of "poop."

A final diet-related technique you can adopt to help with weight management is to drink more water. As you saw, your hydration levels play an important role in how fast your metabolism works. So, the more water you drink, the quicker your metabolism will get. The quicker your metabolism gets, the more calories it'll burn (rather than store them in your body), and the more it'll start dipping into your existing fat reserves to find the energy it needs. It's as simple as that.

What about the more workout-related things you can do to maintain your weight? Obviously, working out regularly is one habit you have to adopt. Another strategy is to mix up your workouts. In other words, combine your strength and cardio workouts and do them together rather than focus on cardio on Mondays, strength training on Tuesdays, and so forth (Schroeder et al., 2019). One way of adopting this practice is to try the lower-impact versions of high impact interval training (HIIT) for about 20 minutes per day.

HIIT sessions combine strength training with cardio. A typical 20-minute session might look a little something like this (Stevens, 2023):

1. Warm Up for two minutes.

2. Do downward facing dog and move to a plank or modified plank and keep the position for one minute.

3. Do one squat set.

4. Do butt kicks for one minute.

5. March in place for one minute.

6. Run on the treadmill for five minutes.

7. Do a set consisting of the following movements:

○ **Glute bridges:** Lie on your back and keep your feet planted on the ground as you lift your hips up.

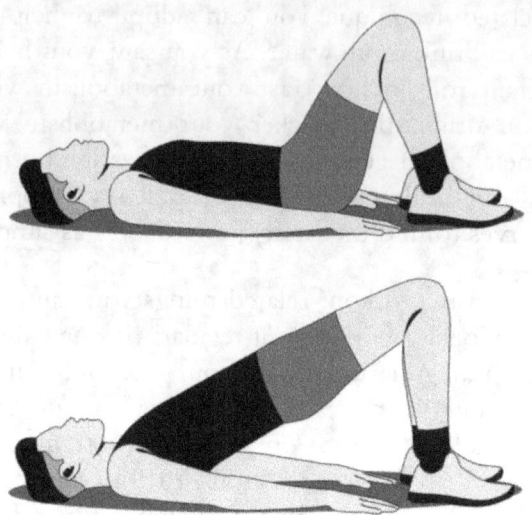

○ **Crunches:** A sort of mini sit-up, except you don't raise the whole way. Instead, raise halfway before going back down and repeating the movement.

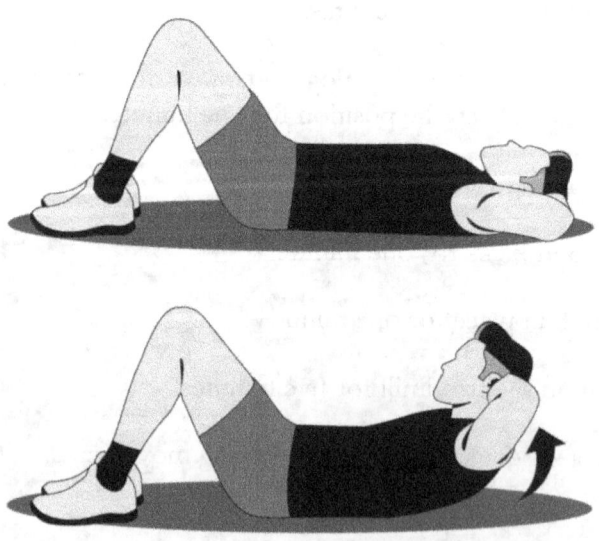

- **Plank holds:** Hold your body aloft by resting your weight on your toes and forearms. Keep your back straight, and don't raise your butt.

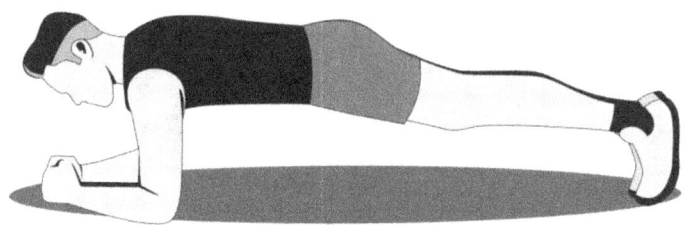

- **Reverse lunges:** Step back with one leg and bend both knees to a 90-degree angle before rising back to your original position and repeating the movement.

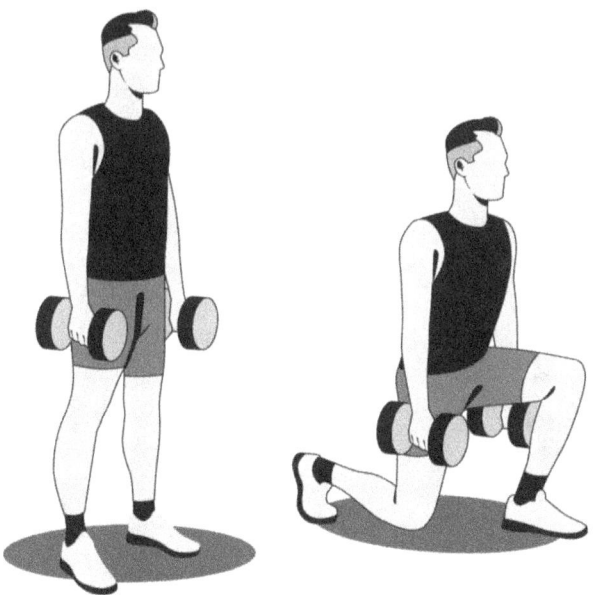

- **Push-ups or modified push-ups:** Rest your knees on the ground and cross your ankles in the air or place your tiptoes on the ground. Then, perform a push-up.

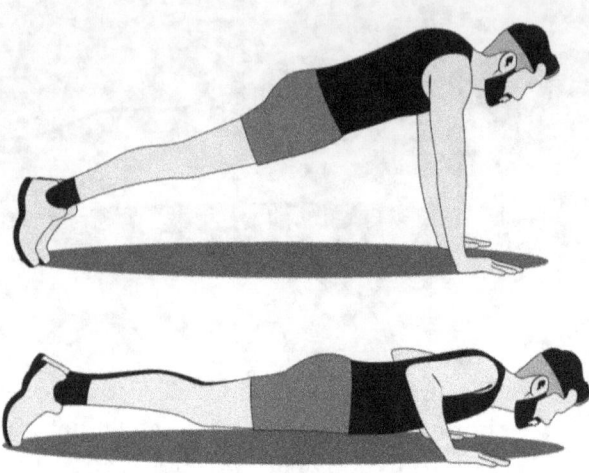

- **Regular lunges:** Step forward and bend both knees at a 90-degree angle before falling back into your start position.

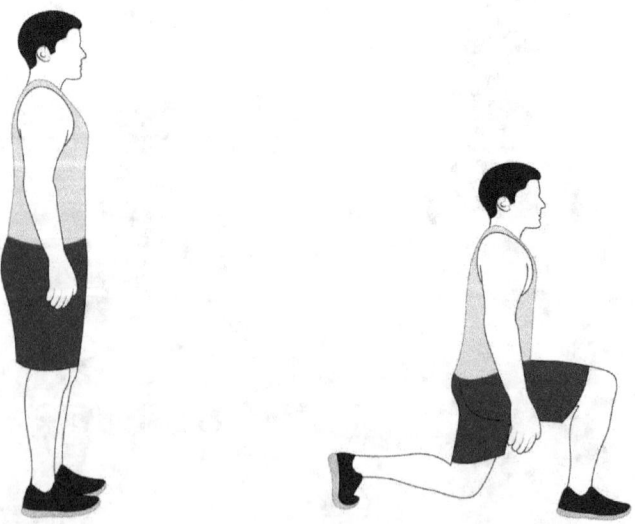

8. Do your cooldowns and stretches.

Regardless of whether or not you give HIIT a try, strength training is something you absolutely need to do for the sake of your muscle strength and because it burns a lot of calories. Your muscles use a lot of calories, as you'll recall. The more muscle you have, the more energy you use and the more weight you lose. Likewise, the more muscle you have, the harder it becomes for you to gain weight (Ritchey, 2023).

Another activity you might try is yoga. Yoga is primarily a balance and flexibility exercise, one that we'll discuss at greater length in the following chapter. Studies have found that practicing yoga for a year makes older adults lose about 0.4 inches from their waist in a year's time (Siu et al., 2015).

There is one last strategy you can actually do to maintain a good weight and healthy body composition, and that's to get all the sleep that you need. Now, you might be a night owl, but even so, it's vital for your health and well-being that you get enough sleep. You see, we have this specific hormone that our body can only produce while we're sleeping. This hormone controls our appetite and how full we feel. When we get enough sleep, we make as much of this hormone as we need. So, we end up with a regular, healthy appetite throughout the day and find that we're better able to tell when we're full. Suppose we don't get enough sleep, though—the exact opposite happens. So, we need at least seven hours of sleep per night. We also need to try to go to bed and wake up at around the same time so that hormone production can be consistent (Frazier, 2021).

## Building a Positive Self-Image and Practicing Self-Acceptance

It's fantastic that you're taking your health seriously and that you want to get into shape. However, that goal doesn't give you permission to judge or berate yourself when you look in the mirror. Wanting to get fit does not mean disliking yourself. The fact of the matter is, no matter what age you are and what you currently look like, you are beautiful and fabulous. You have a strong, wonderful body that has faithfully carried you all these years. You should be proud to have such a miraculous, strong, ever-changing, and beautiful body. Hence, you should not be tearing it down. Wanting to lose or manage your weight doesn't mean doing disliking your current self. It just means giving yourself a bit of a makeover, perhaps with a 90s montage involved, and taking care of your body the way it deserves to be taken care of.

Of course, this is easier said than done, especially as you look in the mirror and see all the changes that have come about over the years. Your first instinct when you look in the mirror might be to criticize these things. You might have the following thoughts: *That part of my body looks disgusting*, or, *I look ugly today*. You do not. It's important that you start changing these thoughts when you have them. If you don't, your self-esteem level will go down. You'll start feeling unconfident and unsure of yourself. In the end, you'll develop a pretty negative view of yourself, which can be damaging, mentally speaking. It can lead to anxiety, confidence, and stress issues and feed into depression.

So, you have to become aware of the negative thoughts you have of yourself. You then have to make a conscious effort to change them. When you catch yourself having a negative thought about your body or how you look, write it down. Now, write down a kinder, more accepting version of it that thought. Repeat this alternate version to yourself, ideally while you're looking at your reflection in the mirror. This activity may seem a little silly initially, but the more you do it, the easier it'll get. After a certain point, you'll start having those positive thoughts more often than the negative ones. So, you'll start seeing your body in a more positive light.

Another practice that can help your positivity and self-esteem is to express your gratitude toward your body. Your body has admirably brought you to this point and carried you through many trials and tribulations without faltering. It has enabled you to do many different things and still continues to do so. Expressing your gratitude will help you develop a more positive body image. It'll also take your focus away from what you can't do or find more difficult these days and place it on what you can accomplish. This will put you in a more positive, optimistic frame of mind, which you'll need to keep going with your workouts and pursuing the goals you set for yourself. A positive mindset, then, is absolutely necessary as we grow not just older but wiser, as we'll see at length in coming chapters. Working on our flexibility and mobility is too, especially since exercises that focus on these two factors help us to accomplish more things that we want and make us more independent in our everyday lives, as the next chapter will demonstrate.

# Chapter 7:

# Flexibility and Mobility

By now, you know that you lose some bone density and muscle mass as you age. But those aren't the only things you lose. You also lose some of your balance and flexibility. This change doesn't become immediately visible when you're 50 or 55, but it does start becoming pretty noticeable at the 60 or 65-year mark. If you make balance, flexibility, and mobility exercise a regular part of your life early on, like in your 50s or even before then, you could prevent the loss of bone density and muscle mass from happening. Thus, when you officially become a senior—with all the discounts that come with it—you can keep yourself from experiencing a dreaded cause of injuries: falls.

Current statistics show that one in four older adults, meaning those over 65, experience falls every year (*Facts About Falls*, 2024). In the US, that number translates to about 800,000 older adults taking a tumble and potentially getting injured as a result. In 2019, 88% of all visits to the emergency room were related to falls; meanwhile, about 319,000 older adults are hospitalized every year for hip fractures, which usually result from falls (*Facts About Falls*, 2024). Things aren't all that rosy for those in their 50s, either. Research shows that people in their 50s are 62.1% more likely to experience a fall than their younger counterparts (Painter et al., 2009).

Our risk of experiencing a fall as we age increases because we lose more of our sense of balance, flexibility, and mobility with each passing year. We lose some of our balance because our joints become more stiff or even damaged as we age, making movement and mobility more difficult (Madison, 2021). We lose some of our flexibility because our spines and tissues lose some of their water content, making them less flexible. The muscle mass loss we experience adds to this change, making us feel weaker and making ordinary tasks harder for us to accomplish (Bowen, 2023). As a result, we lose some of our range of motion and mobility. We also lose a number of neurons, as you'll recall, including ones in charge of managing our motor skills. This process slows down our reflexes as we age, making it harder for us to catch ourselves when we fall and easier for us to get injured (Tracy, n.d.). It's not all bad news, though, because changing all this is well within our power. We just need to make practicing the right balance, flexibility, and mobility exercises a regular part of our routines.

## Stretching Exercises to Increase Flexibility and Prevent Injuries

To start, let's take a look at what flexibility exercises are and why they are effective in preventing falls and injuries. Once you hit 50, you start losing your range of motion, flexibility, balance, and coordination, bit by bit. Stretching exercises are preventative. They make you more flexible and, in doing so, increase your range of motion, mobility, and ability to do whatever you'd like. It makes actions like bending over or reaching for something easier and more comfortable and reduces the risk that you'll pull or strain something while attempting such moves. They make your muscles less stiff and tight. They enhance your body's ability to understand its own position in a room or space. This ability, or sense rather, is called proprioception. You want this sense to be keen because it reduces the risk that you'll trip, knock into something, or knock something over. It also improves your balance.

Thus, flexibility exercises have the added benefit of improving your coordination and balance. They also help lower your stress and anxiety levels, making them great for your mental health and well-being. They promote good blood circulation throughout the body, too, making them very good for heart health and general health alike (MacDonald , 2024).

This overview naturally prompts a question: *What stretching exercises should I be doing at 55?* Before I can answer that query, there's one last thing I need to explain, and that thing is the difference between dynamic and static stretches. As you can probably gather, there are two types of stretches you can and should do. The first type is *dynamic stretches*, which includes motions that are meant to wake up your joints and muscles. Hence, they're perfect stretches to adopt for your warm-up sessions. Alternatively, *static stretches* are moves that place some strain on specific groups of muscles for short periods of time. They only prove effective if you've already warmed up. Without a proper warm-up, their effect remains limited at best. So, they're great stretches to try either immediately after your warm-up or, better yet, during your cool-down session (Brennan, 2021).

Given this new information, let's remedy our earlier question: *What dynamic and static stretching exercises should I be doing at 55?* To start with your dynamic stretching exercises, the ones you might like to incorporate into your workout routine include these examples:

- **Walking lunges:** Lunges are strength training exercises and stretching moves all in one go. To start, stand up straight with your feet at hip-length apart. You then have to step forward with your left foot, making sure to distribute your weight evenly between your two feet. Once you've stepped out, bend both knees at a 90-degree angle. When you achieve this angle, your back knee should be almost touching the floor. If it is, you can rise back up and step back to your original position. Then, you can step out with your right foot and repeat the same move until you can feel a good stretch in your leg muscles.

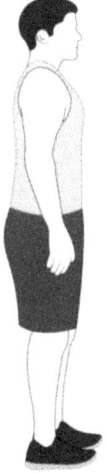
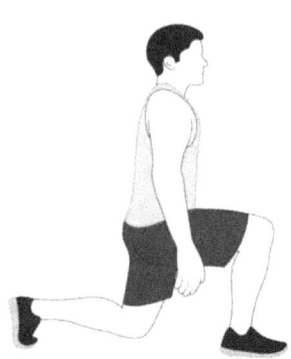

- **Air squats:** Squats are also strength exercises that double as stretching moves when you think about them. To begin, you must stand with your feet shoulder-length apart. Then, perform the squat exactly as you learned in Chapter 4. However, unlike before, you must now hold the squat for a few seconds, keeping your hips in line with your knees and feeling all your muscles stretch before rising back up and repeating the process.

- **Standing quad stretches:** Performing quad stretches requires standing tall with your feet shoulder-length apart and then moving your weight to your right leg. Once you're in this position, you can bend your left leg so that your ankle rises up behind you and grab it. Having grabbed it, you can pull it more toward your butt while keeping your hips facing forward and pushing out your chest. Ideally, you want to hold this pose for 20 seconds before letting go of your foot, lowering it, and repeating the move with your right foot. If you find that you have a tough time maintaining your balance while you stretch your quads, you can perform this stretch next to a wall or with a sturdy chair. You can rest your free hand on this surface, being careful not to give your weight to it so that you have an easier time.

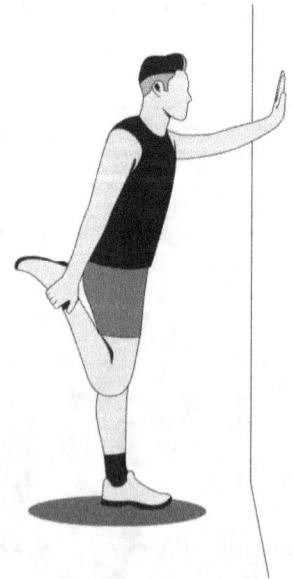

- **Hula-hoop hip stretches:** Hula-hoop hip stretches start with you standing up straight with your feet together for a change. Then, place your hands on your hips and start rotating your hips as though you were spinning a hula-hoop. You'll have to go slower than if you were spinning an actual hula-hoop, but not so slow that it takes ages. You're aiming for an average speed, something between the hare and the tortoise. After 30 seconds, you can start rotating your hips the other way, moving in that direction for 30 more seconds.

- **Chin drops:** Chin drops are great stretches for your neck and shoulder muscles, and they're pretty easy to do. Press your elbows and palms together in front of you while standing with your feet hip length apart. Turn your hands until your palms face your face before moving them to the crown of your head. Next, gently lower your chin, tucking it close to your chest. Be careful not to use your hands to push your chin down, but keep them where they are. Hold the pose for about 10 seconds before looking back up again.

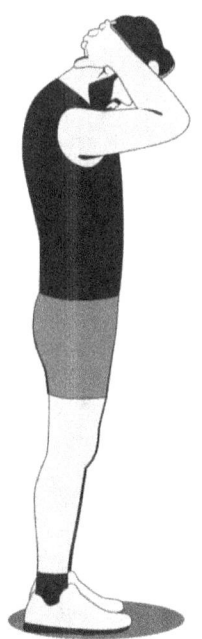

- **Arm openers:** Arm openers are great for your arm, chest, and shoulder muscles. To perform this stretch, you have to stand with your feet shoulder-width apart, then lace your fingers behind your back. Your arms must be relaxed at this point, and your knuckles must face the floor. When you're ready, you can slowly raise your arms up behind you, keeping your fingers interlaced. You should keep going as far back as you comfortably can. Remember, the point here is to feel the stretch, not any pain or discomfort. Once you hit that sweet spot, you can hold the position for several seconds before slowly lowering your arms.

- **Seated shoulder stretches:** Seated shoulder stretches obviously require sitting down on a chair, bench, or another sturdy surface. Sit toward the edge of the chair so that you're getting as little support from the back of the chair as possible, but keep your own back straight. Now, bring your right arm across your chest, almost as if you're trying to point at the opposite end of the room. Support this arm with the other one by placing your hand on your elbow. Gently push and try to bring the inner elbow of your outstretched arm as close to your chest as you can manage, and hold this pose for a few seconds.

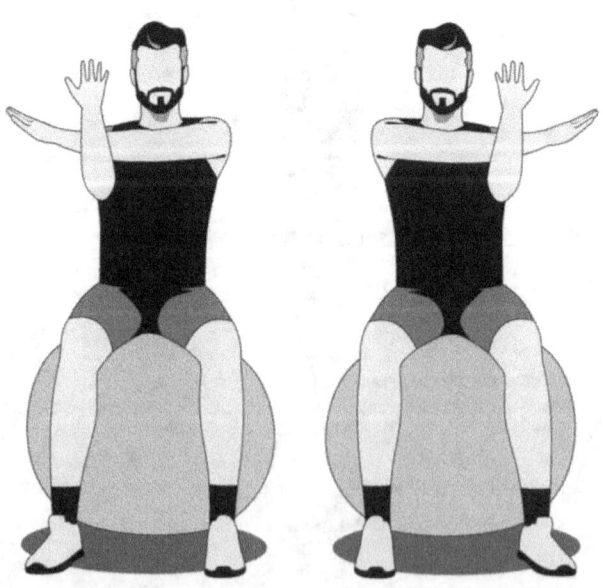

- **Downward dog:** Downward dog, which we briefly mentioned in Chapter 6, is a great full-body stretch to try. Start by getting down on all fours on a firm but cushioned surface, such as a yoga mat. Make sure your knees are hip length apart whereas your arms are shoulder length apart. Now, slowly lift your knees off the floor and straighten your legs without lifting your feet and without moving your hands and feet from where you've settled them. Keep going until you've drawn a kind of upside-down "V" shape with your body. Once you have, slightly lift your heels off the ground, too. Be sure that your spine remains relaxed but straight, as does your neck, and keep the position for a few seconds. Then, slowly lower your heels to the ground and hold that position for a few more seconds before slowly going back to the pose you started in.

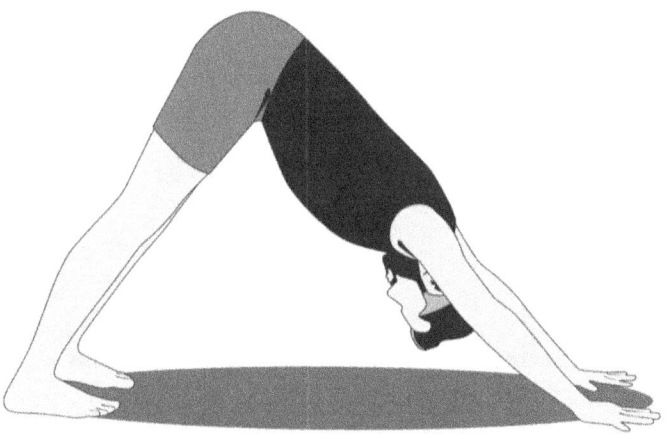

How about static stretches, then? Below, you'll find the best stretching moves to incorporate into your routine:

- **The hamstring stretch:** There are a few different kinds of hamstring stretches you might try, but I'd recommend the seated one because maintaining your balance becomes less of a problem. Start by sitting on the floor with your feet stretched out before you and your back straight. Then, fold in your right leg so that its sole is pressing against your inner mid-thigh. Once you're ready, reach toward the toes of your extended leg without bending that leg and while keeping your back straight.

Grab hold of your foot, if you can, or get as close to it as you can manage. Having reached as far as you can, hold the position for 45 seconds. That's the thing about static stretches. Unlike dynamic stretches, where you should stretch for just a few seconds, static ones require holding a pose for at least 30 and, ideally, 45 seconds. When your 45 seconds are up, pull your hands back, switch your legs, and repeat the same process with your other foot (Asher, 2015).

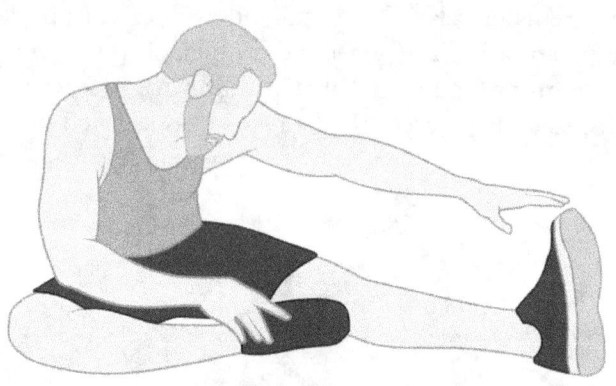

- **The calf stretch:** You'll need a sturdy chair without wheels to perform the calf stretch, except it won't be so you can sit on it. What you'll do instead is to take place directly behind the chair and place your hands on its back for balance. You don't want to give your weight to the chair; you just want to keep hold of it for safety's sake. Keep your feet hip-length apart and in line with one another before stepping back with your left leg, leaving the right one where it is. Keep your back leg straight, and make sure the entirety of your sole, including your heel, is pressing on the ground. Then, slowly bend your elbows so that they jut out to the sides a bit, and bend your front knee slightly. As you do, you'll start feeling a good stretch in your back calf. Hold this position and really feel that stretch for 45 seconds. Then, switch and repeat the same process with your other leg (*Calf Stretch*, n.d.).

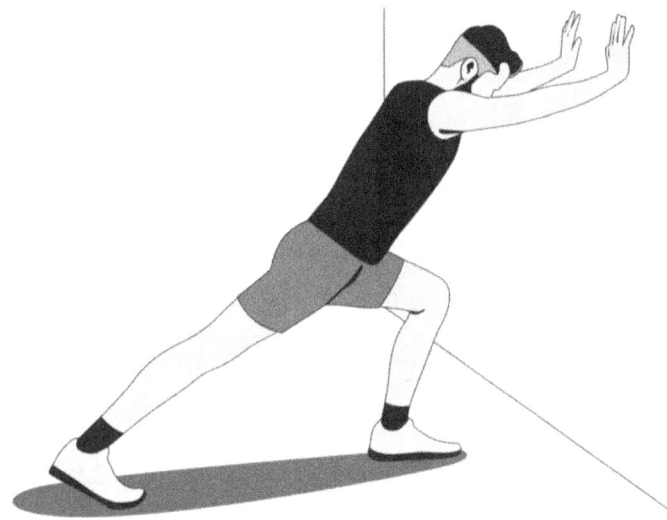

- **The butterfly stretch:** The butterfly stretch is another move that requires sitting down on a firm but cushioned surface, such as a yoga mat. Once you've taken a seat, straighten your back and tighten your abdominal muscles. When you're ready, join the soles of your feet together in front of you, making sure they're lined up with the center of your body. Don't slouch as you perform this movement. Place your hands on the outsides—ordinarily the tops—of your feet. Now, slowly pull your heels toward you while relaxing your knees and trying to get them as close to the ground as possible. You should start feeling a good stretch in your inner thighs. Keep breathing slow and deep while you perform this stretch, and hold the pose for 45 seconds before letting go (Cronkleton, 2019).

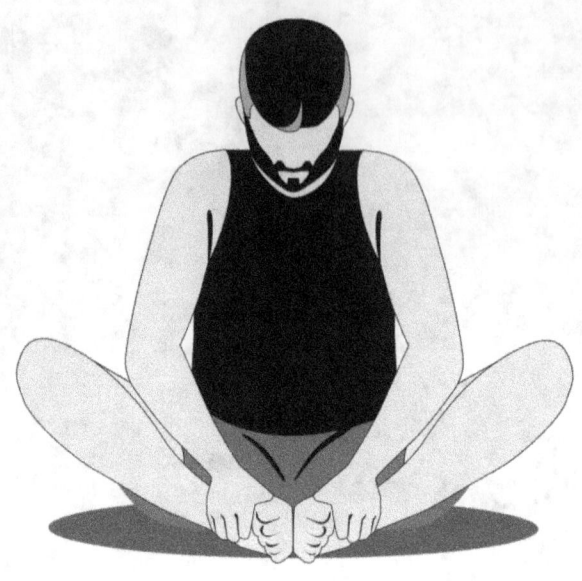

## *Enhancing Mobility for Daily Activities and Active Lifestyles*

As a rule, the more flexible you are, the more easily you can perform your daily activities and lead an active lifestyle. This reason is why stretches, particularly dynamic stretches, should be a part of your workout routine and everyday life. The deliberate movements you perform while doing dynamic stretches are vital for taking your muscles and joints through their full range of motions, preventing them from losing bits of that range of motion and some of their flexibility. As mentioned before, they prepare your body for a thorough exercise session and adequately warm you up.

However, stretching moves, be they dynamic or static, aren't the only type of exercise you can do to enhance mobility for your daily activities and make it possible for you to lead a more active lifestyle. There are, in fact, many other methods you can try on top of that, like foam rolling. Foam rolling is a kind of self-massage method that requires you to use a foam roller or, if you don't have one, some type of ball to apply pressure to certain parts and points of your body. This pressure proves really good at unknotting muscles and relieving any pressure that has built up in your joints.

As you can probably gather, foam rolling is very beneficial for you. For one, it improves your joint flexibility by taking pressure off your joints and greatly relaxing your muscles, especially when it manages to undo any knots that have formed in them. In addition, it takes away some of the fatigue you feel after an intense workout session and relieves you of any painful muscle spasms you may be experiencing. As an added benefit, foam rolling improves blood circulation throughout your body and helps your muscles, which will experience some wear and tear in your workouts, to recover faster afterward (*Foam Rolling for 50+*, 2019).

Of course, these benefits only hold true so long as you know how to use a foam roller properly. The first thing you need to do is to consult your physician. They will be able to direct you and tell you where you need to apply pressure using your foam roller. For example, suppose that you struggle with lower back pain. You might be inclined to use your foam roller on your lower back muscles. That, however, won't relieve you of the aches and pains you're experiencing because lower back pain typically doesn't stem from knotted lower back muscles. This pain stems from knotting or tightness in your hamstrings or hip muscles. Knowing this fact, your doctor will direct you to these regions, and you'll be able to use your foam roller accordingly. Thus, you'll be able to relieve yourself of the pain or discomfort you're experiencing.

If you really want to get into foam rolling, then you're going to have to get a foam roller. Try to get as soft a foam roller as you can. Such a roller will be better for your muscles and joints. Once you've gotten your roller, all you'll need to do is roll it against various muscles and parts of your body. At the start, keep your sessions confined to just 10 minutes. Over time, as you get used to the practice, you can extend the time. You can also start experimenting with the direction you're using the roller in, switching things up when needed.

A word of caution, though: As a rule, using a roller shouldn't be a painful experience. If anything, it should be a pleasing one, where you relieve yourself of the pains and aches you feel and feel better as a result. So, if you experience any pain while using a roller, you should stop immediately. You should also talk to your physician about it to see if you're doing something wrong and to identify any issues you weren't aware of before. After that, based on their recommendation, you can get back into the habit.

Yet another way you can increase your flexibility, range of motion, and balance is by using a resistance band. Resistance band exercises make for great stretching moves. They're also fantastic low impact exercises that can enhance and improve your physical health and well-being and strengthen your muscles. In a way, they can be considered a combination of resistance training and stretching workouts.

The question here, of course, is which resistance band exercises should you be doing? There are a few options for you to choose from, but the best ones, in my experience, include these movements (*10 Resistance Band Workouts for Seniors*, 2023):

- **Calf presses:** Calf presses are the type of exercises you perform while sitting on a sturdy surface like a chair or bench. You want to sit with your back straight and start by planting both your feet firmly on the ground. If you want to grab your resistance band on both ends, lift your right leg up a bit and loop the band's center around it. Next, you want to extend that foot out without having it touch the ground—but keep the other firmly on the ground. The leg you hold aloft must not bend, and its toes should flex and point toward the ceiling. If they are, you can hold the pose for a few seconds before pointing your toes. You can then flex them again and repeat this series of movements 12 times before switching legs and doing the whole thing over again.

- **Bent-over rows:** Bent-over rows are an exercise that you usually do while standing up. However, as you get older, it's recommended that you practice this move sitting down instead. That way, you won't risk losing your balance or overexerting yourself. Place your resistance band in front of a sturdy chair and stand centered with both of your feet. Grab the ends of the band and sit down. Move your feet to the sides a little so that they're hip-width apart. Extend your hands out in front of you and bend forward at your hips, keeping your back straight as you do so. For this movement, you'll need to tighten your abs and squeeze your shoulder blades together. Maintain a 45-degree angle with your body and slowly pull the ends of the resistance band toward your chest. Then, slowly extend your arms back, reverting to your start position. Repeat the movement 12 times, making sure not to disrupt your posture or to pick up speed.

- **Glute bridges:** To perform glute bridges, you'll need to lie down on your back with your hands at your sides, your knees bent, and your feet planted firmly on the ground. You'll need to loop the resistance band around your knees and keep your feet hip length apart at all times. When you're ready, press your palms to the ground and push down on your hands and heels to lift your hips off the ground. Keep going until you form a straight line with your upper body, squeezing your butt and core muscles as you do so. Once you're in position, move your knees to the sides, stretching the band as you go. Slowly take them back to their original position and slowly lower your buttocks to the ground. Once you're fully back to your start position, repeat the move 10 more times.

- **Chest pulls:** Chest pulls are a simple exercise that requires you to stand straight and tall with your feet hip length apart. Now, grab your resistance band on both ends and bring it to the chest level, keeping your elbows bent and tucked into your sides. When you're ready, tighten your abdominal muscles and take a deep breath. As you exhale, straighten your arms and pull the resistance band to the sides without lowering or raising it from the chest level you were keeping it at. As you slowly go back to your start position, breathe in. Then, do another 12 reps.

- **Lateral raises:** Lateral raises are a standing-up move, too. For this one, you'll have to stand on top of your resistance band at its very center and grab it by both ends. You'll need to keep your feet hip length apart. Then, you can fully extend your arms to the sides, pulling the resistance band as you go and keeping your palms facing down as you do so. Your arms should mostly be straight as you do this, but you should bend them ever so slightly. Once you've raised your arms as much as you comfortably can while feeling a stretch, you can slowly lower them back to your sides before doing 10 reps in all.

## Incorporating Yoga or Pilates into Fitness Routines

Two final practices you may want to start are yoga and Pilates. Yoga and Pilates are fantastic practices for those over 50 years old because they significantly improve flexibility, muscle strength, balance, and mobility. To start, a routine yoga practice offers the following additional benefits (Llyod, n.d.):

- Yoga makes it easier for you to fall asleep and helps you get a restful night of sleep.

- It increases and improves your energy levels.

- It lessens chronic pain and makes it far more manageable to deal with.

- It lowers your blood pressure and strengthens your heart and cardiovascular system.

- It lowers stress, anxiety, and even depression.

If you're considering getting into yoga, you should know that you must either do it with an instructor or as part of a class. By doing so, you can ensure you're doing every move correctly, have your instructor fix movements if you're not, and avoid any possible mistakes and injuries. I'd recommend joining a class because then you can turn yoga into a social exercise, too. I'd also suggest trying a few different yoga classes because there are different types out there, and you want to find the one that works best for you.

When you're doing yoga, it's important that you wear breathable and stretchy clothes because the moves and poses involve stretching. Going with a top that won't fall over your head when you bend over is a good idea, too, since certain yoga movements have you doing bends and twists.

The key thing to remember with yoga, though, is to take it slow—especially if you're a beginner. Take just one or two classes per week as you start. Over time, as you gain flexibility and strength, you can up the number of classes you can take. You can also start learning more intense, harder movements, especially as you graduate from beginner to intermediate level.

These same rules apply to Pilates. Pilates is a highly recommended flexibility and balance exercise for older adults. Here are its benefits:

- Pilates increases bone density.

- It improves your posture, making you stand taller.

- It improves your gait and balance, thus lowering your risk of falling.

- It increases your range of motion and mobility.

- It strengthens your muscles and helps you build lean muscle mass.

- It strengthens your immune system, making it harder for you to get sick.

- It decreases back pain by strengthening your abdominal, leg, and hip muscles.

# Chapter 8:

# Sexual Health and Fitness

Contrary to what some people think, older adults don't simply stop having sex when they get older. Odds are you haven't either, but you've probably noticed that some things have changed. Now, most men maintain their sexual interest well into old age, meaning to their 70s and beyond—just ask Picasso. However, as you get older, your testosterone levels start declining. Once you've hit 30, you lose about one percent of your testosterone levels per year! This decline can cause certain changes to your sexual appetite and habits (*Sexuality and Aging*, n.d.):

- It can make your orgasms much shorter than they used to be.

- It can make it harder for you to get or maintain an erection.

- It can result in you needing much longer recovery times after you've ejaculated (to use the medical term).

Of course, your testosterone level isn't the only thing that can affect your sexual health and fitness as you age. Other factors can, too. For instance, certain kinds of medication can alter your hormone levels, including your testosterone level, thus impacting your libido. Medications that treat dementia, arthritis, diabetes, chronic stress, anxiety, depression, and high blood pressure are prime examples. Suppose you are on such medication and are experiencing a lower sex drive or trouble getting aroused or maintaining your arousal. In that case, you should talk with your physician about possible solutions or alternative medication. If your sex drive has fallen as you age, you can also test your testosterone level.

There are home kits you can actually use. If your testosterone level does prove to be low, you can talk to your physician about what you can do to fix it. Your physician might recommend testosterone replacement therapy. You can also increase your libido by incorporating the following tips into your routine (Satchel, 2023):

- Limit your intake of alcohol.

- Get more sleep since not getting enough of it stalls testosterone production in the body.

- Work with a therapist to overcome anxiety and stress issues, as these conditions can be libido-killers.

- Practice mindfulness and meditation for the very same reason as above.

- Eat healthy, balanced meals and exercise regularly.

## Exercises and Techniques for Sexual Health and Pleasure

Exercising regularly is one of the best things you can do to improve your sexual appetite and stamina, as mentioned before. However, certain types of exercises and moves are better for this purpose than others. So, what are the best exercises you can do for your libido's and stamina's sake? Here are some options (Zane, 2020):

- **Forearm planks:** Forearm planks are great exercises for you to make part of your routine because they significantly increase the strength of your core, arm, and leg muscles. They can mimic the missionary position, too. Forearm planks entail resting on your forearms and the tips of your toes while holding your back straight. They use your body's own weight to improve your muscular strength, especially if you manage to hold it for one minute.

- **Push-ups:** Push-ups are a fantastic upper body strength exercise to adopt because they'll increase your stamina for the bedroom. They'll also be a version of the kind of movements you'll perform while in bed. For best results, you should ensure your hands are directly beneath your elbows. This positioning will work your chest muscles. You should also keep your back straight and core muscles tight. You can then bend your elbows as you press down, making sure that your elbows don't bend toward the sides as you go.

- **Upward facing dog:** The upward facing dog move stretches your lower back muscles while opening up your spine and chest and strengthening your shoulders, arms, and wrists. They make you more flexible and stronger—and better able to perform as a result. The flexibility they help you gain allows you to try some new moves or old favorites that you might have forgotten about, too.

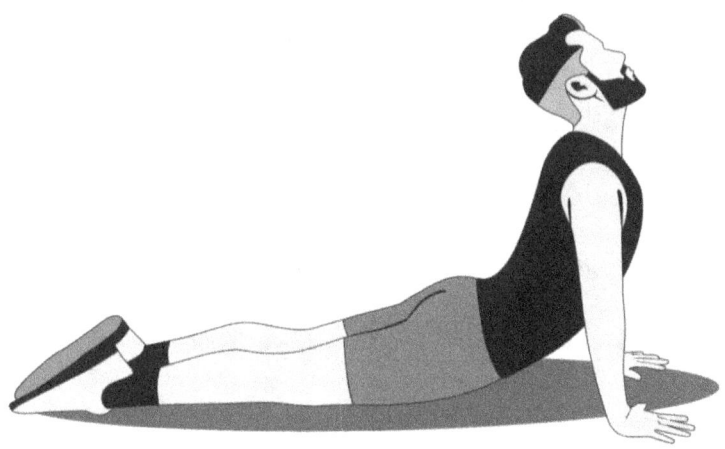

- **Hammer curls with dumbbells:** If there's one exercise you can't go wrong with, it's hammer curls with dumbbells. This move strengthens your biceps, which proves fantastic for any movement where you have to carry your weight with your arms. The move itself is pretty simple. You stand with your feet hip length apart and keep your back straight. You grab your dumbbells and have your palms face the sides of your body.

You keep one hand to your side while the other lifts the dumbbell toward your chest. As you do this movement, you lock your elbow so that only your forearm, not your upper arm, is moving. You stop when the thumb of the hand holding the dumbbell is as near to your shoulder as you can comfortably get it. If it is, you can lower that hand and repeat the move with your other one, continuing on to do 10 reps with each arm.

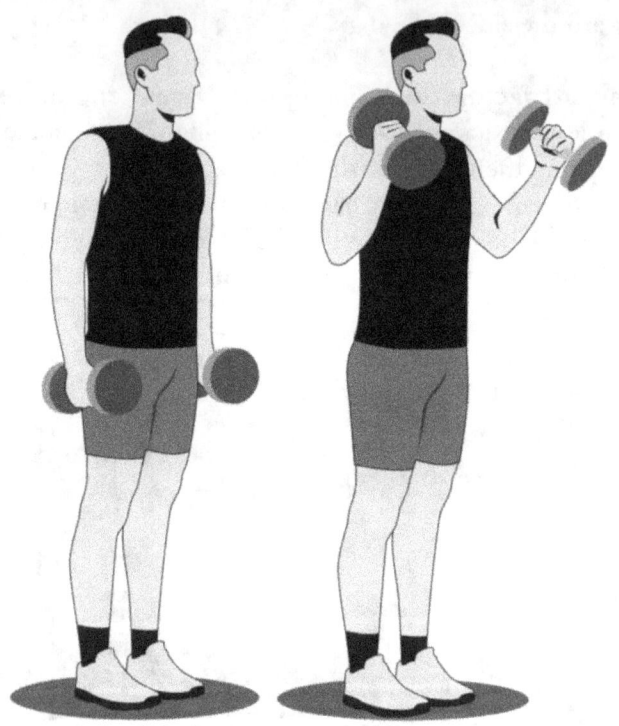

## *Common Concerns for Sexual Health in Older Gay Men*

Aside from dropping testosterone levels and losing some muscular strength and stamina—which you know you can prevent by working out—are there any other concerns older gay men should be aware of where their sexual health and appetite are concerned? Why yes, there are! These sexual health concerns can broadly be summed up with this list:

- pain or discomfort experienced during sex

- erectile dysfunction

- premature or delayed ejaculation

- feeling stressed or sad before or after sex

Now, a number of these issues can be overcome by changing your medication, seeking testosterone therapy, or talking to your physician, as we've covered. Some of them can be solved with exercise, too, especially since it can increase your endurance, strength, and stamina. I mean, let's face it: sex is a strenuous activity. You need plenty of energy and stamina to be able to do it. So, the more you work out and strengthen your body, the more you'll be able to enjoy it. And does your exercise routine make you all the more flexible for it? Well, I'm sure you and your partner will appreciate that, especially as you try new positions.

Speaking of new positions, as fun as sex is, it can get a little... repetitive if you let it. It's easy to fall into a routine when it comes to sex. It's easy to fall into go-to positions, the same way a pro tennis player would adopt go-to moves over the years. While these positions are comfortable and things you know you can do well, having your repertoire consist of them entirely can get quite monotonous. Trying new positions every once in a while should help. So, you might consider changing up your routines. Suppose that you and your partner usually have sex at night before going to bed. Why not spice things up a bit by throwing in some morning sex every once in a while? Alternatively, why not plan a romantic date or getaway for the two of you to rekindle some of your old romance and reconnect with one another?

What if the issue isn't that sex has gotten repetitive or monotonous but that it's become less comfortable or even a little painful? This discomfort can occur because of certain health issues that come with age, like arthritis or back pain. If so, working to find new positions that can make sex more enjoyable would be a good idea. Even doing something as simple as putting a pillow behind your lower back can go a long way. You can also try a side-by-side position, as this will take a lot of pressure off your lower back, unlike missionary.

Another measure to take here might be to pay close attention to your body. When do you feel most comfortable, relaxed, and energized? Those are the ideal times for you to do something strenuous, be it working out at the gym or in bed (Contributors, 2022).

What if your issue, when it comes to sex, is more of an emotional one? What if you're feeling stressed because you feel more pressure to perform now or anxious or sad because you worry that, now that you've grown a bit older, you're not as attractive to your partner as you once were (Mayo Clinic Staff, 2017b)? Those are understandable concerns to have, and we all experience them at one point or another. Worrying over them, however, will not help you. Talking to your partner about them openly and honestly will help, especially since they're likely dealing with the same worries and stress as you. Once you have this intimate, open, and honest conversation, likely two things will happen. First, the two of you will grow closer on an emotional level. Second, you'll be able to work through your issues together, whether emotional or physical, and find solutions that work for both of you. Thus, both your sexual relationship and your emotional relationship will improve.

# Chapter 9:

# Mental and Emotional Health

We briefly discussed your emotional health as it relates to your sexual life in the previous chapter. Now, let's take a closer look at that connection. In this chapter, we'll explore how your mental and emotional health changes as you age, what it might be impacted by, and what you can do to improve it. First things first, though: What exactly is mental health? What is emotional health? How are the two different, and how are they connected?

Your emotional health is an important part of your overall mental health. It can roughly be described as your ability to be aware of, regulate, and cope with your negative and positive emotions. Being emotionally healthy means being able to understand, label, and express your emotions in a healthy way. It means being able to regulate your more challenging emotions, like anger or fear, and keep them from dictating your actions and the course of your day (Brennan, 2021b).

Wait, if that's emotional health, what exactly is mental health? Your mental health can roughly be defined as your ability to cope with the everyday stresses of life, be aware of your own feelings, thoughts, and abilities, learn new things from past experiences, and contribute something to the community that you live in. Simply put, mental health is much broader in scope than emotional health. However, both are necessary for your overall health and well-being, and they're even connected to your physical health.

Before we dive into why your mental and emotional health matters so much, let's get a few facts straight. As of 2021, 5.5% of the entire U.S. population has been grappling with some sort of mental health issue or another (Felman, 2020). That equals about 14.1 million people, in case you were wondering. Sadly, the LGBTQ+ population makes up a disproportionately large portion of this group of individuals. Studies show that gay men are far more prone to having anxiety, stress, and mood disorders than straight men (Rowan et al., 2021). How could that not be the case, considering the stigma, judgment, and discrimination that many gay men are still subject to in their everyday lives? This is especially true for older gay men who have been dealing with such issues for far longer than their younger counterparts. Therefore, studies show that older gay men are more likely than younger gay men and straight men in general to have anxiety disorders or depression (Rowan et al., 2021).

# The Importance of Mental and Emotional Health

These facts are all important to keep in mind because your mental and emotional health matters in more ways than you might think. For example, did you know that having good mental and emotional health is something that improves your cognitive functions and the overall health of your brain? Think about the last time you felt anxious, stressed, or depressed. Were you able to think clearly at that time or not? Were you able to draw logical conclusions, see the full picture you were dealing with, and make sound decisions?

I'm guessing the answer to those questions is "no," and that makes sense because things like stress, anxiety, and depression impact your ability to think and remember things accurately. They also affect, that is to say, lower your problem-solving skills, perceptive skills, and reasoning abilities. Hence, they affect your decision-making skills, too, causing you to make the wrong choices and decisions more often than not (Cleveland Clinic Staff, 2024).

Your mental health also affects your physical health, and it can do so in many ways. For example, say that you're struggling with anxiety. If that's the case, then your anxiety may impact your body in the following ways (Cherney, 2022):

- Anxiety can affect your heart and cardiovascular health by causing your heart rate to be continually high. A high heart rate will wear out your heart muscles and potentially cause heart palpitations. It also increases your risk of having high blood pressure and developing some sort of heart disease.

- Anxiety can cause you to have all sorts of digestive issues, such as nausea, constipation, diarrhea, stomachaches, and even irritable bowel syndrome (IBS). These symptoms occur because blood flow is directed away from your digestive system and toward your limbs so that you can fight or flee from whatever is causing you to feel so anxious.

- Anxiety can weaken your immune system by keeping adrenalin pumping through your body, negatively impacting the immune system's ability to do its job and function as intended.

- Anxiety can lead to respiratory issues by keeping your respiratory rate high and rendering your breaths shallow and rapid. This process can even make the symptoms of asthma, if you have it, worse.

These are just a few examples of what one type of mental health issue can do to your physical health, but I'd say that they're enough to show just how connected mental and physical health and well-being are. I'd also say they demonstrate part of the reason why it's so important that you look after your mental and emotional health.

This is especially true in light of the most recent statistic we have on hand. Currently, one in four older adults struggle with some type of mental health issue, the most common ones being depression, anxiety, and stress. About five to seven percent of all older adults grapple with depression. That may not sound like much, but it translates to up to 2.8 million people, and that's just the over-65 population. Add to that those in their 50s, and that figure skyrockets. Meanwhile, 3.8% of all older adults struggle with anxiety and chronic stress (Brennan, 2021c).

## *Strategies for Managing Stress, Anxiety, and Depression*

So, with mental health issues such as stress, anxiety, and depression being so prevalent and considering how damaging they can be for you, what's to be done? What can you do to manage your stress and anxiety levels? What can you do to combat or even ward yourself against depression? What can you do to keep your mental health strong and to keep yourself resilient, happy, and strong?

If we want to learn how to manage annoying things like stress and anxiety or, worse, depression, then we have to properly understand what they really are. To start, stress is the response your body and mind give to physically or emotionally demanding events. It's a normal bodily response, as long as it remains temporary. The problem is that most of us don't know how to manage stress. As a result, most of us end up wrestling with stress constantly. I don't think you need to know how exhausting wrestling stress can be in order to understand how draining chronic, that is to say, perpetual it can be.

Now, stress is often confused with anxiety, and it's easy to see why. Anxiety and stress have many of the same symptoms. They both cause insomnia and other sleep difficulties. They both can make it hard for you to concentrate on what you're doing, lead to digestive issues, tense up, or make you angry or irritable. Despite these similarities, though, stress and anxiety are not the same. Instead, anxiety is the worry, unease, or fear you feel in a given situation (The Healthline Editorial Team, 2022). That given situation can easily be triggered by stress, which means that, yes, stress and anxiety are connected. Who would have thought?

There is one fundamental difference between stress and anxiety, though: Usually, you feel stressed in response to a specific event or trigger, like your partner texting you, "We need to talk," out of the blue. The same isn't true for anxiety. You can feel anxious anywhere, at any time, for seemingly no reason. If you've ever had an anxiety attack in the middle of a crowded street, you know exactly how fun that can be.

Since stress and anxiety can be so similar to each other, and since they are connected, it shouldn't be surprising to hear that the techniques you need to adopt to manage them are much the same. The first thing you need to do is make sure you get enough sleep at night. When you get stressed or anxious, your body is flooded with two hormones: cortisol and adrenalin. When you get enough sleep, your body starts producing a lot less cortisol and adrenalin. So, these stress hormone levels start going down. This process allows you to keep calm throughout the day and manage your emotions better (*How Does Sleep Reduce Stress?* n.d.).

Another thing that can really help with stress and anxiety is working out regularly. There are two main reasons why. First, when you exercise, your body starts pumping hormones called endorphins into your system. This is a "feel-good" hormone in that it literally makes you feel good. In the athletic world, endorphins are even referred to as "the runner's high," and they very effectively counter and lower your stress hormone levels. Second, exercise actually imitates the physical effects of stress. It makes you breathe hard and fast, increases your heart rate, and makes your palms sweat... Doing so actually gets your body to practice working through those effects. It also helps your body to practice calming down after you've experienced those effects (Mayo Clinic Staff, 2022).

In addition to these strategies, there are three others you can use to manage your stress and anxiety, including meditation, deep breathing techniques, and journaling. Meditation is a scientifically proven way of lowering stress and anxiety levels (Scott, 2018). It's able to do so because it slows down your heart, respiratory system, and even mind, all of which usually get into a massive rush whenever you get stressed or anxious. Meditation works in this way because it triggers your body's relaxation response, just as stress and anxiety trigger its fight-or-flight instinct, so that you may run away from or fight whatever threat you're facing. The problem is that the threats we face today are usually things we can neither run away from nor fight, like taxes, for instance. That means that we can either stay stressed and anxious about them or learn to manage and lower our stress and anxiety in spite of them. Hence, meditation.

Roughly defined, meditation is the art of being fully present. To meditate means focusing on the moment you're in and all the sensations you're feeling within that moment. It means breathing in and out, deeply and slowly, while letting your thoughts drift in and out of your mind. The goal isn't to think no thoughts. Instead, it's to not chase after those thoughts the way you might usually do. This might be a little challenging at first. You might sit still while seemingly doing nothing for an extended period of time. That's perfectly understandable and even to be expected. It's important that you don't get mad at yourself when you catch yourself doing this. What you need to do in such moments isn't to get mad and think things like, "I can't do this," or "Maybe meditation just isn't for me." It's to gently and kindly bring your attention to your breathing and focus on it, relinquishing such thoughts as you do so.

As for how to meditate, you can start by sitting or lying down somewhere quiet, calm, and comfortable. Then, you can close your eyes and start taking deep, slow breaths. As you breathe in and out, focus on your breath. Notice how the air feels as it travels in and out of your lungs. Pay attention to how your diaphragm inflates and deflates. Try to be aware of the feel of the ground or whatever surface you're sitting on beneath you, the temperature of the room, and the soft sounds you can hear. In other words, direct your attention exclusively to the moment you're in. Try to notice your thoughts, too, but again, don't chase after them. Let them come and go as they please; it's something you'll get better at in due time.

Ideally, you want to be able to meditate for about 30 minutes at a single time. However, this might be tricky, especially if you're new to meditation. If it is, then start by meditating for just five minutes. Don't get angry at yourself if you grow distracted or impatient during those five minutes. Instead, keep breathing and bring your mind back to the moment every time your mind wanders off. After about a week, meditating for five minutes will get much easier. Eventually, you'll be able to meditate for longer stretches of time, such as eight or ten minutes. After another week, you can increase it to 15, and then 20. You can keep going on like that until you're able to meditate for 30 minutes straight. For the best outcome, I'd recommend meditating at the same time every day. By doing so, you can turn it into a regular habit. Many people prefer meditating when they first wake up to start the day in a calm, good mindset. Some people meditate right before they go to bed as it helps them fall asleep. I'd recommend either time of day (or maybe even both), though you're free to choose an entirely different time to practice this activity if you'd like.

A second great stress management to try is deep breathing techniques. Now, there are many different deep breathing methods you can try. One of the best ones, in my experience, is called box breathing

(Cleveland Clinic Staff, 2024). Box breathing is a breathing technique often used by the Navy SEALs before they go on an important mission. It's highly effective in lowering stress and anxiety because it can get your heart and respiratory system to calm down in just two minutes. Practicing it is fairly simple, too. Start by taking deep breaths while internally counting to four. Then, hold that breath in while counting to four. Finally, let your breath out slowly while—you guessed it—counting to four. Then, rinse and repeat and keep going for two minutes. When your time is up, your racing heart and shallow, rapid breaths will have calmed down significantly.

A final stress and anxiety relief technique is journaling. When you journal, you can vent, get stuff out of your mind, understand your thoughts and feelings better, and recognize when you're having negative thoughts that get you down. You'll then be able to counter these thoughts and feelings by responding to them the same way you'll respond to a good friend who was experiencing them (Scott, 2023). The great thing about journaling is that you can do it however you'd like, so long as you do it regularly. You can write about anything, be it something you did that day, things that have been on your mind lately, or things that happened in the past that pop into your mind. You can keep your journal entries as short or lengthy as you want, though I'd recommend writing at least two paragraphs per day. That way, you can start getting to the root of your thoughts, feelings, and experiences and start analyzing them a little. As you do this work, you'll get to broaden your perspective about past events, understand your emotions and emotional responses better, and bring some order to your thoughts. This practice will calm down both your stress response and anxiety.

Actually, techniques like meditation, deep breathing, and journaling aren't only good for anxiety and stress. They can be good for depression, too. Depression can best be described as a mood disorder that makes you feel an overwhelming and seemingly inescapable sense of sadness, which can make it hard for you to even get out of bed each day. A great deal of people struggle with depression around the world, but it seems to affect older adults disproportionally. Studies show that 20% of the 65-year-old and up population in the US cope with depression (Harvard Health Publishing Staff, 2018). They also show that depression is often triggered by stress and anxiety, though not always.

Meditation can prevent and reduce depression because it trains your mind to resist and counter any negative thoughts you might be having. That's important because the negative emotions that people struggling with depression are so often mired in are triggered by stress and anxiety. So, the more a person reduces the frequency and intensity of these thoughts, the more they lower their stress, anxiety, and depression levels. The same can be said for deep breathing exercises and journaling.

## *Building Resilience and Cultivating a Positive Mindset*

One of the best things you can do to combat depression, stress, and anxiety is to challenge your negative thoughts and build a positive mindset. A positive mindset not only ensures that you lead a calmer and happier life but also helps you build resilience. Your resilience is your ability to overcome challenges, pick yourself back up when you fall down, and not let the stress of, well, life get to you. But how the heck are you supposed to challenge your negative thoughts and build a positive mindset?

To answer this question, I recommend two things: cognitive restructuring and positive affirmations. Cognitive restructuring is a technique that was developed as part of a therapeutic approach known as cognitive behavioral therapy (CBT). Looking at its name, you might think that it's a difficult technique, but it's not. In fact, it's a simple method, and all you need is some time, a little dedication, and a notebook and pen to carry around with you. You need these latter tools because the technique starts with you writing down a negative thought when you catch yourself having one. Then, you write the more positive or, at the very least, neutral version of that thought. You keep doing this activity every time you have any kind of negative thought. This practice will train your brain to replace negative thoughts with positive ones. As a result, your brain will start performing these steps automatically in time. As time passes, you'll start thinking fewer negative thoughts and a lot more positive ones. That's not to say you won't ever have any negative thoughts, but it is to say they'll be less frequent and less able to affect your good mood (Stanborough, 2020).

The second technique you can try is positive affirmations. Positive affirmations are positive statements about yourself that you repeat every day. They work because of something known as neuroplasticity. You see, your brain is very interesting in that it can't always tell the difference between "fiction" and "reality." This confusion is particularly true in your thoughts. So, when you have a negative thought or imagine a negative scenario about or involving yourself, your brain takes it to be real. It has your body react as if whatever self-image you're creating or scenario you're writing about yourself is real and happening. For example, say that you had a fight with a friend. If you're imagining yourself losing a good friend after that argument, your brain and body react as if that were actually happening. As a result, you may feel upset, afraid, and angry. It convinces you that your friend really will stop talking to you and may even drive you to stop talking to them before they do so. Thus, your negative thoughts and feelings prime your body and mind to experience the negative event you envisioned and, in a way, make sure that it comes to pass.

Positive affirmations hijack the brain's ability to do this. By forcing you to create a positive self-image and craft positive scenarios about yourself, they get your brain to react to those pictures they're painting. This process generates a lot of positive emotions and primes your body and mind to take positive action. Thus, it increases your belief in yourself and your appreciation of yourself. They also make it easier for you to take the actions you want to ensure the optimistic scenarios you envision actually unfold.

For this to be the case, you have to practice positive affirmations every single day. I'd recommend doing this activity in the morning and in front of a mirror so you can start your day in a good headspace. You also have to write the right kinds of positive affirmations for them to work, which means you have to follow certain rules. Your positive affirmations must adhere to these guidelines (Raypole, 2020):

- be in the present tense

- be specific to you

- be realistic and actually achievable

- be about things that are in your control directly

Affirmations must be in the present tense so they feel more real for your brain and help you to take advantage of neuroplasticity better. They must be specific to you rather than generic because then they'll be directly in line with your goals and values, making them all the more meaningful to you. They must also be realistic because otherwise, they're neither achievable nor believable. If you've never worked out a day in your life, for example, then writing an affirmation about how you're going to win the marathon that's going to take place next week isn't going to help you. Writing one about how much stronger you're going to get and how much your stamina and endurance will increase thanks to your efforts will help. Finally, your affirmations must be about things directly under your control. Thinking back to the marathon example, winning the marathon isn't necessarily something under your control because you cannot control the performance, endurance, age, and stamina levels of the other contestants. You can, however, control your own endurance and stamina levels since you can increase those through regular workouts. Hence, writing an affirmation about winning the marathon won't be a good idea. Writing one about your endurance and stamina will be since they're things under your control and since your affirmation will motivate you to push yourself a bit more in training and improve more than you could have imagined in these areas.

# Chapter 10:

# Aging Gracefully and Mindfully

Having discussed practices like meditation, positive thinking, and deep breathing techniques in the previous chapter, we would be remiss not to dive into mindfulness. Mindfulness is a mental skill—I'd say it's also an art form. The practice focuses on being fully present and aware of the present moment. The thing about aging is that many of us are very resistant to it. By that, I don't mean that we can physically resist aging—though we technically can to a degree with things like Botox and hair dye—but only to a degree. I mean that we show a lot of mental resistance to it.

As we spot the signs of aging in our bodies, whether physical or otherwise, we become upset or even angry. We look in the mirror and start disliking what we see, as if aging is synonymous with ugly, which—let's be clear—it isn't. As clichéd as it may sound, every age has its beauty, which means that you should be able to look in the mirror and acknowledge the person standing before you as beautiful and fabulous. You should be able to take pride in the person you see standing before you. But being able to do so requires two things. The first is to accept the inevitability of aging and even embrace it, which mindfulness can help you with. The second is to show yourself the self-care and self-love you need and deserve. The question is, "How?"

## Embracing the Aging Process With Grace

There's a term for approaching aging with mindfulness: positive aging. Positive aging works exactly as it sounds. It entails adopting a positive approach to aging. This approach naturally means changing the more negative beliefs you hold about getting older and embracing positive ones instead. It's important that we do so for several reasons. For one, embracing positive aging will obviously help us like ourselves more, leading to happier lives. For another, studies show that holding negative beliefs about getting older increases our stress and anxiety levels and can even lead to depression. Such beliefs make us feel more isolated from the world, impact our health negatively, and even shorten our lifespan, at least according to some studies (National Institute on Aging Staff, 2020).

Meanwhile, other studies show that holding positive beliefs about aging does the exact opposite. It increases your happiness, life satisfaction, and desire to live (Chopik et al., 2018). These studies also show that positive beliefs about aging make you more resistant to illness and better able to recover when you do fall ill. They push you to be more proactive about your health, which means they make it easier for you to do things that are good for your health, such as eating healthy, balanced meals, working out regularly, and practicing self-care—something we'll talk more about momentarily. On top of all that, positive beliefs about aging lower our stress levels, which keeps stress from turning chronic, thereby sparing us the chronic health issues that such stress can lead to.

## The Importance of Self-Acceptance and Self-Love

Of course, your ability to reap these benefits depends on your ability to adopt positive beliefs about aging. The first thing we need to do to embrace this mindset is to practice self-acceptance and self-love. Practicing mindfulness techniques such as meditation and journaling will help, and so will cognitive restructuring and positive affirmations, particularly if those affirmations are about your aging self. Another measure that'll help with self-acceptance, which is the ability to accept yourself as you are, is celebrating your own abilities.

We all have our own unique skills and abilities—including you. You shouldn't minimize or dismiss them. After all, they are part of your strengths and are likely among the things you enjoy doing. They are part of you and part of what makes you unique. So, why should you dismiss your own uniqueness? Why should you dismiss your own self?

A great way to celebrate and remind yourself of your abilities and achievements is to write them down (Cassata, 2021). Go ahead and make an entire list of your strengths. You can remember them and discover ones you didn't realize you had by asking yourself, "What do I enjoy doing?" "What have I gotten better at over the years?" and "What am I really good at?" You can then write your answers down. Odds are that you'll be surprised at how many different things you discover.

Why stop at just writing, though? Why not try new things and activities to discover new strengths, interests, and hobbies? Despite what some might say, it's never too late or too early to discover new strengths. It doesn't matter if you're 17, 70, or somewhere in between. You can always try things you've never tried before and end up learning something about yourself in the process. So, go ahead and sign up for new classes. Try activities with your friends or family that you have never tried before. Volunteer in new places and go to new events. You probably won't fall in love with every single new thing that you do, but you might with one or two. For example, if you've decided to give golf, crochet, or baking a go, you might realize you have a penchant for these hobbies. So, you might start doing them more and more. In the process, you will celebrate skills you didn't know you had and ensure you keep leading an active lifestyle, even as you age.

That's another thing that's vital for self-acceptance, self-love, and graceful aging. Part of the reason many of us dislike getting older is that we hold this mistaken belief that we'll have nothing to do or won't be able to do anything once we age. However, this isn't true. Well, it's only as true as we make it. If you believe that you can't do anything as you age or that you have nothing to do, you won't try anything new. You won't engage in your old hobbies or go out to do things. So, you'll turn your beliefs into self-fulfilling prophecies. If you believe otherwise, though, then you'll be more enthusiastic, willing, and eager to both partake in hobbies you already enjoy doing and try out new ones. Thus, you'll prove to yourself you really can engage in life more, even as you age, creating yet another, though this time more positive, self-fulfilling prophecy.

One strategy for embracing self-acceptance, self-love, and aging is to practice gratitude, particularly gratitude toward your aging body (Cooks-Campbell, 2022). Gratitude is a very powerful tool. It's something that can quickly remind you of all the blessings in your life, thereby preventing you from getting swept away by negative thoughts and feelings. It can generate a lot of positive feelings instead. This process is doubly true when you practice gratitude for your body. Yes, your body has gone through many changes over the years and shows signs of aging, like gray hair and wrinkles. However, that body has been through a great many things and still managed to carry you all the way here.

Yes, you may have some aches and pains now, but your body is still strong and flexible enough to help you do all sorts of things. What's more, it has the potential to be more flexible and stronger, so long as you eat right and work out. These are all things for which you should express your gratitude. To do so, I'd suggest keeping a gratitude journal and writing at least five things you're grateful for today. Perhaps you're grateful that you're healthy and able to go about your daily life. Perhaps you're grateful that your muscles are getting stronger because of your strength training efforts. Perhaps you're thankful your feet were able to carry you a significant distance today as you completed errand after errand. Perhaps you're grateful for your eyes, which still enable you to take in the beauty of the world, even if your eyesight has become slightly less sharp over the years.

Whatever the case may be, write it down and do so every day. By doing so, you'll get to focus on all the positives about your body rather than things that are more negative and unchangeable. You can take this process a step further by making sure to engage in activities that promote self-acceptance and body positivity, such as working out. These activities will drive home your body's capabilities, strengths, and value even more. It'll make it possible for you to embrace your body and yourself, showing yourself the love that you deserve.

In the meantime, there are a few other things you can do and some habits you can adopt to embrace aging. One is to make a point of learning new things. We already mentioned that trying new activities is a good idea—one that can help you notice strengths and hobbies you weren't aware of before. Learning new things by taking classes, reading, and doing other similar activities is an extension of that, one that keeps your mind active and engaged. Keeping your mind active and engaged as you age is very important because this keeps your brain strong and sharp. In other words, it keeps your brain healthy. Studies show that people who are lifelong learners are much less likely to develop conditions such as Alzheimer's than people who are not (Celias, 2023).

The pursuit of learning, then, can keep your cerebral muscles strong and sharpen your cognitive skills. It can also boost your mood by increasing your self-esteem, which will naturally increase the self-love and self-acceptance you show yourself. As an additional benefit, seeking to learn new things is often something that widens your social circle. Going to a class or workshop, for example, usually means meeting like-minded individuals. Over time, these individuals can turn into friends, thus broadening your social circle. More friends usually mean more people to spend time with, doing all sorts of things. So, by meeting new people, you can adopt a more active lifestyle. You can, therefore, be more engaged in your own life, as well as more mobile, something that will contribute to your physical health as well as your mental health.

## *Mindful Self-Care and Self-Compassion Practices*

If there's one last thing you can do to embrace aging, it's to practice self-care and self-compassion regularly. Self-compassion is your ability to show compassion toward yourself. Self-care is an extension of that. Self-care is a catch-all term that includes anything and everything you do for your own physical, mental, and emotional health and well-being. It's a term that's misunderstood by many because there's an incorrect but pervasive idea floating around that self-care is a selfish thing. It's not. In fact, nothing can be further from the truth.

Imagine that your partner is having a rough day. You want to be there for them, supporting them and making their day better. That's very admirable and just what you'd expect of a loving relationship. Now, consider the following scenarios and decide under which conditions you'd be better able to take care of your partner. When you're tired, emotionally drained, and running on fumes, or when you're well-rested, feeling good, energized, and strong? Obviously, the answer to that question is the latter scenario, and you can only achieve that state if you are able to practice self-care and show yourself some self-compassion on a regular basis.

The next question we need to ask is obvious: How can you start practicing self-care at age 55? What counts as self-care, and how can you do more of it? First of all, anything you do to take care of yourself physically, mentally, and emotionally counts as self-care. Some self-care activities change from person to person. After all, self-care is about self-enjoyment, and you and I might enjoy entirely different things. For example, you might find playing chess to be eminently enjoyable and relaxing. I, however, might find it really boring and frustrating. At the same time, I might really enjoy watching old Disney movies. However, you might dislike Disney movies and find them childish.

Which of these activities, in that case, counts as self-care? Put simply, they both do. One is self-care for you, and the other is self-care for me. Self-care activities can change from person to person, depending on their tastes, interests, and hobbies. What if you're unsure of what your interests and hobbies are, though? What if you've grown so accustomed to taking care of others over the years that it has been a long time since you practiced your hobbies or have done anything that you particularly enjoy for just yourself? If that's the case, then it's time to start exploring a bit. Think back to your past. Which activities did you really enjoy before you got into this self-destructive pattern of ignoring your wants and needs? What were you really good at? Make a list and decide on at least three things you'd like to get back into. Then, actually start doing them.

At the same time, start working on another list. This time, list your interests. What subjects, areas, and activities sound most interesting to you, even if you've never done them before? What would you like to have tried at least once in your life? Once you're done with this list, go over it slowly and pick three you'd like to try. Then, either find a class on the activity you've chosen that will allow you to try it or get whatever supplies you need to be able to try it at home. Then, simply start doing whatever it is you've chosen.

By getting back into old hobbies you've parted ways with and trying different things in an attempt to discover new ones, you can start practicing self-care. However, self-care isn't just about hobbies, interests, and activities that you like. It's also about giving your mind and body the rest, nourishment, and care that they need. This is why certain acts of self-care are universal and unchanging for all. For example, making sure you get enough sleep every night is most definitely an act of self-care since it ensures your body and mind get the rest they need. This is especially true for older men. You might have felt fine enough running on three hours of sleep when you were 35, but at 55, that's not a good idea. In fact, it's something that your body and mind can't really take and something that's sure to tire them out very quickly.

The same logic applies to eating healthy, well-balanced meals. Eating food is a way of supplying your body and the various organs and systems it's made of with the nutrients needed to function properly, as you saw before. Making a point of adopting healthy eating habits is something that can only benefit you. Hence, it counts as an act of self-care. Working out regularly by doing strength training, flexibility, and cardio exercises does as well. These exercises increase your muscle strength, joint flexibility, and stamina, as previously discussed. So, they increase your mobility and ability to live independently as you age. When considered in that light, working out can't be thought of as anything other than an act of self-care.

This logic can actually be applied to anything and everything you do that ensures your physical and mental well-being. Take annual check-ups, for example. Annual check-ups can be annoying, but they must be a part of your life. From your blood pressure to your cholesterol, thyroid, and blood sugar levels, everything must be checked over. That way, if anything is slightly askew, it can be discovered early on before it gets to be a major problem. Once you hit 50, you should start getting prostate exams on top of all the regular tests and checks. You should similarly get colon exams. After age 50, men are at an increased risk for Hepatitis C, so that should be among the things your healthcare provider should keep an eye out for as well (Pierce-Smith & Watson, n.d.).

One key thing you should always do as part of your self-care activities is make time throughout your day for rest. I don't just mean sleep. I mean rest and relaxation time taken throughout the day. A lot of us tend to be rest-averse because we think it's synonymous with laziness. It's not. In fact, rest is a very necessary part of a healthy and productive lifestyle. This is because getting rest throughout the day is something that gives your body the time it needs to recover from the physical and mental exertions it goes through. Ensuring your body is well-rested helps prevent falls, accidents, and injuries. Rest also replenishes our energy levels throughout the day, which makes us more productive at whatever it is we choose to do. At the same time, it gives our muscles the time they need to recover after strenuous workout sessions. Our muscles use this time to knit themselves back together and become stronger. Our immune systems use it to get stronger, too. Meanwhile, inflammation levels throughout the body go down when we rest, along with our blood pressure and stress levels. So, rest is very good for our heart and cardiovascular system, too.

Rest isn't just good for our physical health, either. It's essential for our mental and emotional well-being. When we take regular breaks throughout the day, we give our minds, which tire themselves by running all sorts of errands and computations, the break they need. This allows us to replenish our mental reserves, which in turn increases our focus and energy, sharpens our memory, and improves our various other mental faculties. The fact that rest lowers our stress levels helps, as stress and anxiety steal from cognitive functions such as concentration and memory. Stress also feeds into our negative emotions, making it more difficult for us to regulate them. Getting rest prevents this and makes it easier for us to manage our emotions, challenging or otherwise.

So, how much rest should we be getting throughout the day? How much is too much, and what's not enough? The answer to these questions partly depends on how busy a lifestyle you lead and how much you work. Assume you work or that you lead a somewhat active lifestyle. There are two rest techniques that I'd recommend you try as part of your self-care routine. The first is called the Pomodoro Technique, and no, it does not involve spaghetti pomodoro, though it can be used if you want it to.

The Pomodoro Technique is a time management method that has you working or concentrating on whatever it is you're doing for 25 minutes straight before taking a 5-minute break. Then, you work for another 25 minutes before taking another 5-minute break. You repeat this cycle four times. Then, you finally take a longer break, one that lasts between 15 and 30 minutes. Doing so gives your brain the reprieve it needs to re-energize, refocus, and keep operating at peak conditions.

What if you don't like being interrupted so much? If so, you can give the Ultradian Rhythm a try. The Ultradian Rhythm is a method that's based on the idea that our bodies operate best in cycles of 90 to 120 minutes. That means that we're the most productive and that we do our best work when we work for that length of time. However, when that time is up, our productivity, energy, and motivation levels start decreasing. So, the Ultradian Rhythm dictates we should work for 90 to 120 minutes straight, then take a 20-minute or so break to recharge (*The Importance of Rest*, 2023). If we do, we'll be raring to go for another work session once our rest time is up.

# Chapter 11:

# Social Support and Community

We all need someone to lean on—or so the famous lyrics go. The sentiment is incredibly true, even if it does ring just a little cheesy sometimes. You realize how true it really is when you discover the positive effects of social support and community on your physical health, mental health, and even fitness level.

Studies have found that having a strong social support system is crucial for warding us against things like depression, isolation, and loneliness. These studies, which literally took brain scans of their subjects, found that individuals who have the social support they need in life have altered brain functions. As a result, they are at a lesser risk for all sorts of conditions, such as heart disease, other cardiovascular issues, and alcohol use and addiction. Studies show that social support literally expands people's lifespans (Reblin & Uchino, 2018). That finding means that, yes, if you have people you can depend on in your life, you'll typically live longer.

That's not all. It has also been found that social support is essential for your ability to cope with stress and lower your stress levels. This is because people who have strong support systems are able to share their stress with the people within those systems. They are thus able to regulate their stress and anxiety better. Turns out, social support is essential in dealing with stress, and it can even help manage the symptoms of stress-related conditions such as post-traumatic stress disorder (PTSD) (Cherry, 2023).

# The Role of Social Support in Fitness

Strong social support systems offer two additional benefits that will actually support your decision to start a workout routine and stick with it. The first of these benefits is that it supports healthy decision-making. In other words, having social support is something that pushes you to make healthier decisions for yourself and your mental and physical well-being.

So, people with social support tend to eat healthier and more balanced meals, exercise more often and regularly, smoke and drink less, get the daily and nightly rest they need, and take better care of themselves in general. This improved decision-making occurs because of several reasons. First, having social support makes someone feel more valued and happier, naturally increasing their willingness to do all they can to live as long as they can. Of course, that translates to picking up habits that are good for them, like working out and maintaining a healthy diet. Second, having social support often means having people in your life who cheer you on and sometimes even join in on your efforts to lead a healthier lifestyle. These people love you, after all, and want the best for you. So, doesn't it stand to reason that they would support you as you start working out and encourage you to do all you can to become the healthiest version of yourself?

What might this encouragement and support look like in that case? Well, suppose that you live with your partner, and you told him you'll be leading a healthier life from now on. You shared your new meal plan with him, walked him through the exercise routine you meant to stick to, and confided in him your intention to cut back on your drinking habits. Your partner was pleased because he wants you to be healthy, strong, and well—of course, he does! After your discussion, your partner went out. He came back with bags of groceries bearing all sorts of healthy ingredients so that you could immediately start your new meal plan. He even offered to cook the meals with you and told you he'd be eating the same food you'd be eating from now on! That's exactly what the two of you did that night, and it was great.

The next day, you woke up to head to the gym. You found your partner in the kitchen and also wearing workout clothes. Your partner smiled and told you he'll be your workout buddy from now on. So, the two of you headed to the gym. As you worked out, you kept encouraging, challenging, and pushing one another to do your best. By the time you were done, you were exhausted but content. The two of you went home for a well-deserved shower with smiles on your faces. Thus, you fell into a rhythm. Both of you started eating more healthily, working out, and cutting back on less healthy habits such as drinking. At events and get-togethers you went to, you prevented one another from slipping or going overboard. On days when you felt lazy and tried to come up with all sorts of excuses as to why you couldn't work out— the old "I can't find my headphones, so I can't go to the gym" excuse comes to mind—your partner pushed you to do so. On days when he didn't feel like working out, you did the same for him.

The days went on in this fashion, with the two of you pushing and encouraging one another. After a while, working out and eating healthily became habits. You no longer had to think about them and convince yourself you needed to stick with these decisions. They've become reflexive parts of your life, you see. Now, I'm not saying that this can't happen if you don't have a workout buddy or social support. But I am saying that it'll be a lot more difficult in that case. Social support will aid your healthy living efforts because the people in your support system will actively help you stick to your goals. They'll be your cheerleader or workout buddy, someone to vent to when things get tough, and someone to turn to for advice. Essentially, their presence, words, actions, and encouragement will make it easier for you to stick to your fitness decisions for the long term rather than give them a try for a few days before giving up.

That's just the first benefit social support has to offer in your fitness journey, though. Another thing that must be taken into account is that social support helps you stay motivated. The thing about working out is that it's a slow process in some ways. Many people start working out and expect to see immediate results in the form of a shrinking belly and already bulging muscles. However, things don't work out that way. That's not to say that you won't make any progress a week into your fitness journey, but your progress will probably be less visible than you want it to be. That experience can be disheartening. It may cause you to take a look in the mirror, get upset, and decide that working out just isn't working out for you.

I mean, at least it would if you didn't have a solid support system by your side. You see, having a support system means having someone to talk to about your expectations, thoughts, feelings, and disappointment. So, when you look in the mirror and fail to see the progress you were hoping to see, you might go to a good friend who knows you've started working out and share your thoughts and feelings with them. That friend can then comfort you and remind you that progress takes time. They can remind you that seeing visible results will take a few weeks and encourage you not to give up. They'll draw your attention to what you've achieved through dedication and effort thus far and what more you can achieve. This dynamic will help you fix your admittedly unrealistic expectations. It will refocus your mind on your efforts and push you to keep going. It can, therefore, increase, rather than decrease, your motivation level, making sure you remain dedicated to your fitness journey.

Having a solid social system can further increase your motivation if at least some of the people in your social circle are from your fitness community. They'll understand what you're going through, doubts and all, better than anyone else (Hernandez, 2023). They've been through and maybe are currently going through exactly what you're experiencing right now, after all. Hence, they'll be able to offer you the support you need and share what worked for them when they started doubting their own efforts and ability to keep working out in this manner. Furthermore, they'll be able to help keep you accountable for your fitness goals. They'll be able to do this by working out with you, doing friendly check-ins to make sure you're persisting with your fitness journey, and even having others at your local gym or wherever it is you're working out doing friendly check-ins on you.

Your fitness community will also be able to add to your motivation by sharing expert tips and advice that can help you overcome specific barriers to fitness—more on that in the next chapter—and progress faster in various areas. They'll be able to share their considerable expertise with you, help you figure out the answers to any questions that may have been bugging you, and help you fix any mistakes you may be making, thus ensuring that you're able to avoid a fall, accident, and some type of injury, such as a sprain. They'll be able to compare their workout plan with yours and help you optimize your plan. Similarly, they may seek your advice, and sharing your expertise with them will no doubt make you feel valued and like you've made more progress than you might have thought.

If there's one last benefit to fitness communities as social support systems, it's that they make working out into a more social endeavor, as in the "working out with your partner" example. Belonging to a fitness community makes working out into a social activity. Suddenly, you're not just working out. You're spending time with old friends and making a few new ones at the gym and in the classes and courses you take. That can be an incredibly motivating thing, especially if you're looking to lead a more active lifestyle in the first place. As you start spending more time with these new friends, your relationship with them will grow closer and stronger. Before you know it, you may end up with really valuable friendships, going as far as to say, "Where have you been all my life?" and laughing when your new friend responds with, "Here at the gym."

## Building A Strong Support Network

With all of these benefits in mind, there's an obvious question to ask: How do I build a strong support network for myself? The first thing you need to understand about support networks is that you can build one at any age. Don't get me wrong; I hope you already have a few people in your network that you can turn to for social support, like a partner or a few really good friends. Don't worry too much if you don't, though. What you don't already have, you can always build through some time and effort.

First, start by going over your social contacts and social life. Who are you closest with? Who do you rely on for social support when you need it? Who relies on you in turn? Do you talk to these people as much as you should? Do you actually turn to them when you need help, or do you fixate on trying to solve everything for yourself? How much do you spend with the people in your life? Who reaches out to whom more often, you or them?

Answering these questions is important for two reasons. First, you can take a proper inventory of the people in your support network and clearly see who you're close with and can rely on. Second, you can determine whether you're nurturing your relationship with these people as much as you should. For example, if you have people in your social network but are always coming up with some excuse whenever they try to meet up, then you're likely not spending enough time with them. Assuming these are people you want to keep in your life, that's something you probably want to fix.

So, you've taken inventory of your social network and determined who's in your support system, how close you are with them, and how much time you really spend with these individuals. Now what? Well, now, you focus on actually spending time with them. Close, reliable, and supportive relationships and friendships aren't built overnight. They take a lot of time, care, and dedication. So, the more quality time you spend with the people in your life, the closer your relationship will become. This isn't just true for the initial stages of a friendship or relationship. It's true for all its stages. As a rule, you always want to make time for your friends. By that, I don't mean you should drop everything you're doing, work and all, the moment a friend calls just to chat about nothing. I do, however, mean that you should spend time with them regularly. I also mean that you should be there for your friends if they call you for a little support and help. Remember, relationships are two-way streets. They're about "give" as much as they are about "take." If you want your friends to support you when you need it, then you should support your friends when they need it as well. It's as simple as that.

Let's go back to the concept of time for a moment. Yes, you want to make time for your friends and the people you care about. However, you want that time to be a quality time where you actually share things with one another and build trust. That's not to say you shouldn't ever attend a silly comedy show together. But you should also make time to really talk, sharing your feelings, thoughts, experiences, and more with one another. In other words, you should be vulnerable with the people in your life if you want to build trust with them and grow closer to them.

The thing about vulnerability is that it invites further vulnerability. When you share personal goals or intimate feelings with friends, you essentially tell them, "I trust you with this precious thing." That trust makes your friend feel valued. It makes them want to both reciprocate your trust and share their vulnerabilities with you. It makes them want to support you when you share something challenging, too. Now, of course, I'm not saying you should talk about your parents' excruciating divorce from when you were a kid with a stranger you just met on the street. But you can share this with a friend you're already close to if you want to. If you're going to be friends with that stranger, you can start sharing some things with them, too, but you'll start small. Say that you and this stranger decided to meet for coffee after you were done working out. You went to a café and started chatting about your day. Why not tell him about your day? Why not share some minor things about yourself with them? After all, that's how you get to know people.

Suppose your coffee chat went well, and you decided to keep hanging out with this friend. Over time, as you grow closer and get to know them better, you can start sharing more and more things with them. You can start being just a little vulnerable with them and see where that takes you (Craig, 2019). They can start doing the same thing in turn. Thus, you can begin building a trusting and truly caring relationship with one another and will be able to support one another through challenging times as you grow closer.

There's an important point to remember: Just as you can't make easily visible progress in the form of bulging muscles after working out at the gym for just one week, you can't build trusting, supportive, and close relationships with people overnight. Relationships take time, dedication, and effort on both your parts. Consider this scenario: You have a friend who you're always making time for, but they're never making time for you. Can you really consider them a friend? What if you're always there to support them when they're going through something, but they're never there when you need support? Is "friend" the right term for this person in this case? Probably not.

That's another reason you should take inventory of your social support system. Sometimes, we end up letting people into our closest group when they don't actually deserve to be there. Sometimes, our relationships with people change, yet we hold onto them for the sake of memory and nostalgia. We really shouldn't do either one of these things. We should allow people who deserve to be included in our social support system. I don't mean you should cut people out of your life the moment they become unable to offer you support, of course. We're all human, and we all go through all sorts of things. A good friend who's typically very supportive of you might go through a rough patch in life and, therefore, require more support sometimes. They may also be less able to support you during such times. That's perfectly alright and acceptable. In fact, that's an excellent opportunity for you to be there for your friend. What's unacceptable is keeping "friends" in your social support system when they're never willing to offer you support or when they don't care to spend quality time with you. Such people can be acquaintances but friends. Let's be honest: You're much too valuable to give that title to those who don't deserve you.

## The LGBTQ+ Community for Fitness Activities

Obviously, not everyone in your social support network is going to be a part of your fitness community. However, some people will and, more to the point, they should be. Better yet, just as you go about building a support system for yourself, you should build a fitness community, too, ideally one that is LGBTQ+.

Having a fitness community to rely on is generally important, but it's especially so for LGBTQ+ people, no matter their age. This is because people in the LGBTQ+ community can face a lot of added challenges when trying to work out and get fit. For one, they may struggle to find a gym or space to work out in where they feel welcome. For another, having spent long years not feeling like they belong, they may experience a great deal of self-doubt in traditional gyms and workout spaces. This challenge may be especially true for older LGBTQ+ people, and it can be a severe roadblock to them on their journey to get fit.

Seeking out workout spaces for LGBTQ+ people specifically can help. Building spaces for them, if your area lacks such a space, can too. By that, I don't mean you should start your own LGBTQ+ gym, though it's great if you can—and more power to you. You might consider forming a workout group, perhaps over Facebook, with other

LGBTQ+ people. That way, you can meet up with this group regularly and exercise together. You can support one another on your individual journeys and get all the help you need as you work to meet your own fitness goals.

Now, you don't have to go to the gym with your LGBTQ+ community. You can do any number of different activities together. You can, for example, take different classes together, like yoga, Pilates, or dance (*Benefits of LGBTQIA+ Team Sports and Group Exercise*, 2024). You can swim or do different team sports together, too. The point here isn't necessarily which activity you do. It's that you do whatever it is as part of your community, and doing so will enhance the feeling of belonging that you experience while working out. Your community will also be a safe space for you, affording you protection from things like homophobia, which you unfortunately can still experience in the outside world. Within this community, you'll feel safe and accepted, which will make it even easier for you to keep going with your new fitness regime.

# Chapter 12:

# Overcoming Barriers and

# Challenges

By now, it should be clear that growing older is no barrier to fitness. In fact, it should be abundantly clear that you *can* and *should* work out regularly as you age. However, there might still be a tiny voice in the back of your head coming up with all sorts of reasons as to why you can't work out. These excuses can easily stop you from starting your fitness journey if you let them. Likewise, they can get you to give up on your fitness journey after you've already begun.

I hope you noticed my use of the words "if you let them" in the previous paragraph. I used this language because whether you allow such excuses and reasons to actually become barriers for you as you work to get fit is entirely in your hands. You have the power to overcome whatever barriers or challenges you face along the way. All you need to do is know how to roll up your sleeves and start climbing over them one by one.

## Identifying Common Barriers and Challenges

Let's be honest: There is no end to excuses as to why you can't work out. If you try hard enough, you can come up with all sorts of reasons why you shouldn't go to the gym today. As you get older, you don't even have to try that hard. The excuses, or rather, barriers and challenges to working out, as we'll call them, just present themselves to you. However, these barriers and challenges aren't insurmountable. If you know the right strategies and methods you need to employ to overcome them, you can practically skip over them. With that in mind, what are the most common barriers to fitness as we age, and how can we overcome them?

## *Fear of Injury*

Fearing injury is one of the most typical barriers to fitness as we age, and it's easy to see why. As we age, our bones and muscles get weaker. We also start having trouble with our balance and flexibility, and hurting ourselves becomes more possible as a result. At the same time, recovering from injuries is tougher. That being the case, we want to do all we can to protect ourselves and make sure we remain strong and injury-free. Imagine thinking that it would be very easy to get hurt while working out, so exercise becomes the first thing you cut out of your life. Ironically, this does not help you to avoid injury. If anything, it speeds up the rate at which your muscles and bones weaken, which makes it even easier for you to fall or get into some other accident, hurting yourself in some way (Barone, 2024).

So, while the fear of injury may be understandable, it is slightly illogical. When done right, working out won't increase our risk of getting injured. Instead, it'll decrease that risk. Now, obviously, the keywords there are "when done right." If you're doing yoga poses incorrectly without realizing it, then you might strain or sprain something. If you wear clothing that is too loose for the gym, it may get caught on one of the workout machines, causing you to fall. If you're doing jumping jacks at home on top of a slippery rug, then I hate to break this to you, but you're definitely going to slip.

The trick to avoiding injury while working out is to take the necessary safety precautions. Put on the proper clothing and shoes before you start working out. Make sure you're working out on a sturdy surface that is free from clutter underfoot that might cause you to slip. Work with an instructor or at least in front of a mirror so that you can be absolutely sure you're maintaining good form. Take each movement slowly, especially if you're doing strength training and balance-flexibility exercises—don't rush through them. Pay close attention to your body and stop immediately if you feel any pain or discomfort other than the typical muscle burn that comes with exercising.

So long as you take these safety measures, you should be able to start working out and get into a nice fitness regime without any issues. As you keep working out, your muscles and bones will become stronger, and your balance and flexibility will improve. This will lower your chances of experiencing a fall and suffering an injury. In the event that you do get injured, working out will make it possible for you to recover more quickly than you otherwise would have been able to. Remind yourself of these facts every time the voice in your head says, *But what if I get hurt?* as you're getting ready to work out. Then, start your exercise routine as planned and keep going.

## *Health and Mobility Issues*

Just as many people think working out as you age is a bad idea, plenty more think they can't exercise if they have any pre-existing health or mobility issues. Both groups are equally wrong. To start with health issues, let's say that you have some heart issues. Does that mean you can't work out? Contrary to what you may think, it doesn't. In fact, it's doubly important that people with heart conditions work out because regular exercise, as we've seen, strengthens the heart and cardiovascular system. This means that exercise helps with heart disease. It lowers things like cholesterol and blood pressure, strengthens the heart muscles, and reduces any symptoms of heart disease you may be dealing with (Chen, 2022).

To be clear, it isn't just people with heart disease that should make a point of exercising regularly. People with other conditions—such as those with respiratory conditions like asthma, metabolic conditions like diabetes, and chronic problems like rheumatoid arthritis—should, too. Exercise can help with all these conditions and more. Now, of course, this doesn't mean that people with specific health conditions should do whatever exercise they want. There are certain exercises that people with specific conditions will have to avoid. Likewise, there are specific exercises they will have to do. For example, as a rule, people with heart conditions shouldn't do exercises that involve heavy lifting. They should, however, definitely do cardio exercises to strengthen their heart (*Exercise for Heart Failure*, 2022).

Health issues aren't actually a barrier to working out, so long as you find out which exercises you must do and avoid in light of what health issues you're dealing with. The same goes for mobility issues. Consider this concept: If mobility issues were insurmountable obstacles to exercise, then the Paralympics wouldn't exist. True, having mobility issues does mean certain exercises aren't ideal or doable for you. For example, if you have bad knees, you want to avoid running since that movement is hard on your knees. Similarly, if you're in a wheelchair, running isn't going to be an option for you. So, you'll just have to find exercises that work for you. If you really do have bad knees, then swimming might be a great option. If you are in a wheelchair, then upper body resistance training exercises and even group sports like wheelchair basketball may be in the cards.

## Not Fit Enough

Another prevalent barrier to working out is that you're just not fit enough for it. This argument is a little confusing at first, but it starts making sense when you look at it through the lens of body image issues. If you've never worked out before or if you haven't worked out in a long while, you may be a little reluctant to start doing so now. You may think that your body won't be able to handle it since your stamina and endurance levels will be very low. You may also be hesitant to start working out because you feel like you'll be judged at the gym, particularly if you don't already look fit. Being of a certain body type, you might feel like everyone will stare at you, judge you, or maybe even laugh at you as you try to work out. Unwilling to go through such an experience, you may give up on the idea of working out altogether.

If you're dealing with the first hurdle here, meaning the idea that you don't have the stamina and endurance necessary to work out, think again. I mean, obviously, you're not going to suddenly get the endurance level and stamina level of a marathon runner overnight. However, start working out regularly and keep at it, and you'll develop that stamina and endurance level over time. That's how working out works. Remind yourself of this fact every time you feel this objection arise within your mind.

What if you're dealing with the fear of judgment? Well, there are a couple of different things you can do in this case. First, try meditating a bit before going to the gym. The truth about gyms and other similar workout spaces is that everyone is there for themselves. Absolutely no one is there to gawk at other people and judge them. So, regardless of your current fitness level and body type, very few people, if any, will be looking at you as they exercise. More likely, they'll be so focused on their own burning muscles and getting through their own exercise routine that they'll barely register you. If they do, it'll be for a millisecond, and odds are, their thoughts won't be unkind. They may even find you admirable when they take in the fact that you're exercising to get into shape in your 50s.

If you still have trouble overcoming this barrier, try to remind yourself of these facts. Why not get a workout buddy? You can take some of the pressure off by going to a fitness place with such a friend. You'll have someone to rely on and who can help motivate you to keep going when you feel your worries and anxiety rising up. Still hesitant? How about starting your workout journey at home? Don't get me wrong, working out in a gym or by taking classes can be great and very social, but who says you have to start there, especially in the age of the internet? If there's one thing I've learned during the pandemic and the subsequent lockdowns, it's that exercising at home is more than possible. You just need to find the right YouTube video or Zoom class. This can be a great way of raising your stamina and endurance level and getting into shape a little before venturing out into the gym or other similar spaces for the first time.

## Not Enough Time

Another common reason why people say they don't or can't work is that they don't have the time for it. Now, it's perfectly understandable if you don't have the time to work out for an hour straight every day. Here's the thing, though: You don't have to work out for that long, as long as you meet the 150-minute per week workout requirement. It really doesn't matter how short your individual workout sessions are— they can even be just 15 minutes. Exercise for 15 minutes in the morning and 15 at night. Would you look at that? You've already worked out for 30 minutes today. Repeat that for five days in a row, and before you know it, you've completed 150 minutes of exercise already. Who would have thought?

You also don't have to work out in the mornings and nights if you don't want to. When you exercise is entirely up to you, just as long as you do. The basic point I'm trying to make is simple: You have the time to work out (American Heart Association Staff, 2018). You just need to review your schedule to determine *when* that is. My advice? Once you have figured out the perfect time, schedule it. Set reminders so you don't skip them. On insanely busy days, when you can't spare the time to go through your regular exercise routine, take advantage of the waiting times you have here and there. Waiting for the laundry to be done? Do some sit-ups in the meantime. Waiting for your food to cook? Time to stretch.

## Don't Have Anyone to Workout With

Having a workout buddy can be highly motivating, as you know, especially if you already struggle with motivation. What if you don't have anyone to workout with, though? What if your partner, friends, and family members aren't interested in fitness? That can be pretty demotivating, especially if they tempt you to skip a day.

A great way to overcome this barrier is to share your fitness goals with the people in your life and ask them for their support. Invite them to join you if they'd like. If they do, then great! You'll have a workout buddy, and the two of you will be able to motivate each other and hold one another accountable. If they don't, they'll at least be able to cheer you on and help make things easier as you persist with your fitness program. In the meantime, start looking into classes, courses, and group exercises you can join. By doing so, you can surround yourself with people who want to get fit, like you, and turn exercising into a new social activity. You can make new friends and, thus, transform your workouts into things you actually look forward to rather than a chore.

## Don't Have the Resources or Equipment You Need

What if you don't have the resources you need to join a gym? What if you don't have the equipment you need to do some of the workouts we discussed, like dumbbells? That's perfectly understandable, but again, it's not the insurmountable barrier you may be making it into. Let's say you don't have the resources you need for a gym membership or to go to a class. Who says you need one to work out? You can find plenty of free online classes and courses at various community centers if you look for them. You can go for walks, go cycling, or do anything else that does not require paying a monthly fee to work.

And if you don't have the equipment? Well, you don't necessarily need them. For one, strength training exercises can be done using your own body weight. In fact, if you're new to strength training, using your own body weight rather than physical weights is probably a good idea at first. If you really want to use weights, though, you can find something to use in their place. For instance, milk jugs are a great alternative for dumbbells. Laundry detergents, backpacks filled with heavy things, and laundry baskets can be wonderful substitutes for barbells. Really, there is no end to the alternatives you can come up with, so long as you use your imagination a bit.

## Strategies for Staying Motivated and Overcoming Setbacks

Now that you know how to overcome all those barriers and obstacles, maintaining your motivation to work out shouldn't be a problem, and you shouldn't encounter any setbacks, right? Oh, if only that were the case. The problem is that motivation can be a fickle thing. You might start out your fitness journey immensely motivated, only to find that you've completely lost your will to keep going just a few weeks in. This is especially true when you hit a fitness plateau.

When you first start working out, your body isn't used to strenuous activity. As a result, you start getting some pretty tangible results early on in your workout journey. After a certain point, however, your body will get used to this activity level. So, you'll seemingly stop getting results. If you're trying to lose weight, it will become harder at this point. So will building muscle (Cronkleton, 2022). This is what's called a fitness plateau, and coming across yours can be pretty demotivating if—say it to me—you let it.

So, how do you not let it? For one, you remind yourself that this is a phase, and it too shall pass. No plateau is endless, after all. For another, you'll have to adjust your workout strategy a bit to overcome this plateau a little more quickly. Switching up your workout routine is a good strategy. This can include the order in which you do things, the specific exercises you do, and the intensity at which you do them. Alternatively, you can start working out for a little while longer or more often if you have the time.

Another way to overcome a plateau and keep it from demotivating you is to try new activities and exercises. This will get different muscle groups working in your body and in different patterns, and the change-up may prove to be just what your body needs. Alternatively, you may try something called progressive overload. Progressive overload is a method that requires you to increase the frequency and intensity as you work your muscles. The idea behind it is simple: If you're no longer making progress with your exercise routine, then increase its intensity. You can do so by lifting heavier weights, doing more reps and sets, or adding additional exercises to your existing routine.

Taking these measures should help you overcome your fitness plateau and keep your motivation levels up. The keyword is *should*. If they don't immediately work, don't fret. Keep pushing forward, and also, consider talking to a professional, like a trainer at the gym, to get their advice. Sometimes, nothing beats a bit of observation and personal experience.

Hitting a fitness plateau isn't the only reason your motivation levels might lag. There might be numerous other reasons. One might be that you don't actually enjoy the workout you've chosen for yourself (Better Health Channel Staff, 2012). For example, consider going to the gym. Some people love going to the gym, while others really dislike it because they find it repetitive and boring. This latter group of people find it really difficult to stay motivated enough to keep going to the gym day after day. Honestly? I don't blame such people. My advice for them, though, isn't that they quit working out. It's that they find an athletic activity that they actually enjoy doing. To be clear, this is my advice to anyone who is starting their own fitness journey. How long do you think you can keep doing something you dislike or find really boring, even if it is really good for you?

Another reason why your motivation levels might be dropping is that you haven't set realistic fitness goals for yourself. Not setting realistic goals means not being able to meet those goals. Not being able to meet your goals means finding fault with yourself and losing motivation. So, if this problem is what you're struggling with, do a quick re-evaluation of your current fitness level. Ask yourself whether the goals you've set for yourself are really realistic for that level. If the answer to that question is "no," then rewrite your goals. When you're done, come back to your workout session and try again. Pretty soon, you'll start meeting the new goals you set for yourself. As you do, you'll start feeling pretty motivated.

Just so you know, you can maximize this effect by keeping track of your progress. Suppose that one of your goals is to run a mile in nine minutes. For reference, the average 55-year-old man who doesn't work out all that much can run a mile in 12.08 minutes. Your starting speed, let's say, is 12.48 minutes. So, you start training, and after a week, you shave that time down to 12.23 minutes. Then, you shave it down to 12 and then to 11. As you keep advancing, you keep a record of your progress, and you keep this record until you achieve your goal of running a mile in nine minutes. When you do, you feel an immense sense of satisfaction. You also feel this satisfaction each time you enter a new milestone in your record book while working toward your goal and anytime you glance through it. So you feel more motivated to keep going each time you pick up your notebook. Simple, right?

## Dealing with Ageism and Discrimination in Fitness Spaces

Remember how worrying about your body image can keep you from working out? Well, worrying about your age and about facing discrimination because of your age *and* your sexuality can do so as well.

Again, while these are not insurmountable problems, they are important ones to discuss.

Let's kickstart that discussion by focusing on your age. Fitness spaces, such as gyms, are thought to be "young" spaces in that you don't see a lot of over 55-year-olds in them. This can cause you to hesitate a bit. The old worries about standing up can eat away at you, keeping you from working out. In this way, ageism can be rather self-imposed. Reminding yourself that everyone is at the gym for themselves and that no one is looking at you is very important. Journaling and talking to friends who are similarly into fitness and close to you in age can, too.

What if ageism isn't a self-imposed barrier for you, though? What if it's a palpable thing in whatever workout space you go to? In other words, what if you're discriminated against for your age? As a gay man, you're probably, and sadly, no stranger to discrimination. So, you likely have some tools at hand that you know to turn to in such circumstances. One is to obviously raise awareness. Talk to the people in your fitness space, the people in charge of it, not whatever idiot is bothering you, about this. Discuss how the community, including the trainers, in that space can be trained to help support fitness practitioners of a certain age. In other words, use your voice and advocacy to raise awareness among those around you.

While you're at it, try going to your fitness space with friends who are around your age. This way, you can start challenging people's perceptions a bit. You can also have additional support and backup in your fitness space if you need it and are worried about ageism or homophobia, for that matter.

Now, part of you may be thinking, *This is exhausting. I just want to work out. I don't want my workout session to turn into yet another battle over my sexuality or age.* You're absolutely right to think and feel this way, and perhaps the fitness space you've found isn't the best fit for you. Looking into other, more inclusive spaces may be a good idea. These days, there are plenty of LGBTQ+ spaces you can take advantage of. There are even quite a few LGBTQ+ gyms and workout spots you can try. If your area lacks such a spot, why not start your own workout group, as suggested before? By doing so, not only can you ensure you get to exercise in a comfortable place, feeling that you really belong, but you'll also have the social support you need through your fitness journey right by your side.

# Chapter 13:

# Staying Fit for the Long Haul

Getting fit and into shape is a fantastic goal to set for yourself in your 50s. However, committing to staying healthy for the rest of your life is an even better goal to have—even though it's a harder goal to commit to. This is because turning exercise and healthy eating habits into lifelong habits is a challenge. There comes an inevitable time when you have to skip a workout because you're sick or because something truly urgent comes up. When this happens, going back to your workout routine suddenly becomes a lot harder than it used to be, especially if it's not just the one workout you've skipped. The same goes for maintaining your healthy eating habits; once you fall off the wagon the one time or hop off it temporarily because you're celebrating your partner's birthday or because it's Pride, going back to healthy eating becomes a challenge, even if you know the tastiest recipes.

How exactly are you supposed to overcome this situation? How can you make sure you stick to a healthy lifestyle for the rest of your life? How do you get through those days when working out is too hard or eating healthy is too difficult?

## Strategies for Preventing Relapses and Staying Committed

If you haven't been able to work or eat as healthy as you normally would have for a while, the first thing you have to come to terms with is that this is perfectly okay. No human being can ever be perfect because no human being is a machine. Even machines can't be perfect all the time, so don't expect such perfection from yourself. A good way to approach this idea is to consider your workout journey just that: a journey. Journeys don't always unfold at the same pace. They sometimes slow down or pick up the pace. Sometimes, you take a few breaks along the way, too, and that's alright. Don't beat yourself up for slowing down every once in a while or for taking a break or two—intentionally or not. Instead, commit to getting back into the flow of things once your break is over.

If it really has been a while since you last worked because of an illness, a vacation, or some other reason, start by making a plan to recommit yourself to your health and wellness journey. Remember how you created a workout plan when you first embarked on this journey? Create a new plan for yourself now, one that will ease you back into your old workout routines. The key word there is "ease." Here's the somewhat annoying truth: It's okay if you haven't worked out for a few days, but that will usually mean your muscles will get a little weaker, and your conditioning level will go down a bit. In fact, the longer you spend not working out, the more this will happen. So, if you haven't worked out for, say, the past month—that must have been some vacation!—then your muscles will be just a little weaker, and your stamina and conditioning will be lower than they used to be. As a result, you may not be able to lift as much or work out as long as you used to. Getting mad at yourself won't help you. Acknowledging this fact, planning for it, and getting back to work will help.

With that in mind, make a plan for the next two to four weeks. Don't start thinking beyond that period, at least not for now. During those initial weeks, work for two to three days a week. You'll feel the urge to commit to more, but don't do so quite yet. If you do, you'll overtax your body and over-exhaust yourself. So, you'll likely conclude that you just don't have it in you anymore and give up (McCoy, 2016).

Once you've worked out a few times a week for a few weeks, you can start upping the ante. Eventually, you'll be able to work your way back up to your previous workout schedule. More importantly, you'll be able to stick to it. This, of course, will be a lot easier for you if you actually set achievable goals for yourself. Things will improve if you set SMART goals that are appropriate for your current fitness level—not your fitness level from a month or two ago. If you set goals that aren't good for your current fitness level, then you won't be able to meet them. You'll probably get upset, and quitting your workout routine altogether will become infinitely easier as a result.

A great way to ensure you're setting the right goals for yourself while getting back into fitness is to test your current fitness levels, just as you did when you were starting your workout journey. This will give you a full and accurate picture of what you're currently capable of rather than have you focus on what you used to be able to do or what you're supposed to do. Don't worry, you'll get there again. You just need to work your way back to it, and that takes a little bit of time and effort, and there's nothing wrong with that.

What if the problem isn't that you haven't worked out in a while? What if you don't want to work out today? What if you have to drag your feet to the gym, the court, or wherever you may be working out? First of all, don't berate yourself in such moments. Trust me, everyone has them, even pro athletes. You can adopt a few strategies in this case, and you wouldn't know it, but they're methods that professional athletes actually use. Some recommend committing to much shorter workout sessions on days you just don't feel like exercising. If you think about it, even a few minutes will do in such circumstances. That's what Tunde Oyeneyin, a Peloton instructor, recommends you do on days filled with workout dread, anyway (Holmes, 2022).

Another thing you can try on days like this is exercise snacking. No, this does not mean jogging to the corner doughnut shop for a double-glazed treat. It means fitting bite-sized exercise sessions into your day. Making a point to climb the stairs rather than take the elevator is one way of doing this. Another way is to carve just eight minutes out of your day and choose three or four exercises that you'd do in your normal workout routine—eight minutes is doable, right? Once you've done that, you can set your timer for 30 seconds and do those exercises. You can then set your timer again so that you can take a 20-second break. When that break is up, you can repeat your exercises and keep going like that until your eight minutes are up. This mini-exercise session will be very useful in getting you over your exercise hump and prevent you from taking that one off day that unspools into you never exercising again.

If you really want to push yourself to exercise on a day you just don't feel like it and would rather laze around instead, you can try some motivational tactics that might get you up and moving. One of these tactics is to wear an outfit that makes you feel good. Obviously, this outfit must be workout-appropriate. You should be able to move comfortably and not get caught on anything that could make you fall. But who on earth said that you couldn't still look fabulous in your workout clothes? Take some time curating your workout outfits, a process you should enjoy, given that you have a fantastic fashion sense. Choose outfits that are as glam as they are comfortable, rather than the mustard-stained t-shirts that some gym bros tend to sport. These outfits will make you feel really good about yourself while getting you in the mood you need to be to work out.

Playing some good music and creating a playlist that you can work out can also help. In fact, blasting a few songs from that playlist before you start working out can be a great idea. By doing so, you can get caught in the emotions that a piece of music taps into. You'll have an easier time when the time finally comes to get started with your warmups and exercises. This method will be even more effective if you let go and dance a bit before your workout. This will get your blood pumping a bit and serve as an effective way to warm up. Who knows? Perhaps you'll decide that you want to make your dance moves a part of your current warm-up routine.

A last measure you can take to sustain your motivation and remain committed to your workout journey, even on days when you really don't feel like working out, is to focus on your future self. We are often far too focused on the present or the immediate future when we're working out or otherwise trying to keep healthy. While being present is typically a great idea, focusing on a more future-oriented vision when you're working out is a better one. Because here's the thing: That future, healthier, fitter version of you? That's the whole reason you're working out the way you are. However, when you get too focused on the day-to-day, or when you're having one of those days when working out just seems too tiring, too boring, too much work, too "insert adjective here," you quickly lose sight of that vision. Thus, you lose your motivation a bit. You lose even more of it if you're not seeing any immediate results from your training. Thoughts such as "This isn't working" and "Why am I even doing this?" start crawling through your mind. As time goes by, these thoughts accumulate until you conclude, once again, that exercising just isn't for you and walk away.

So, how exactly can you focus on your future self and prevent this from happening? There are a couple of ways you can go about this, and setting long-term health and fitness goals is one of them, so long as those goals remain SMART. A second way you can go about this is to use visualization exercises. Visualization is a psychologically proven method that even the best professional athletes in the world regularly use to achieve the results they want, be they fitness or success-related. It's a method that's highly effective in helping you achieve whatever you want to achieve because it takes advantage of something known as neuroplasticity in your brain.

You see, your brain cannot really distinguish between "real" and "fictional." So, when you imagine something happening, your brain takes it to be real. If you imagine something stressful, it gives the order to release stress hormones in your body, such as cortisol and adrenalin, and your body starts displaying the typical stress-related symptoms, like a racing heartbeat and shallow, quick breaths. But what if you imagined something much more uplifting, relaxing, and motivating? Then, your brain would release more calming, feel-good hormones. This would help you to think more positive, uplifting, and motivating thoughts. In other words, it would help you to get into a positive mindset. Because of this, working out would suddenly become easier. Working out would also become easier if you were to visualize the workout you were about to do before you did this. This would trick your mind into overcoming the resistance it was showing to exercising that day, allowing you to actually get started when you're ready.

As you can see, visualization can be a highly effective tool for increasing your motivation to work out and committing yourself to your fitness journey. This only holds true, though, if you know how to properly visualize the outcomes and processes you want. So, what are you supposed to do? For starters, try to choose a calm, quiet moment and place to start your visualization practice. That way, nothing around you will be able to distract you. Next, close your eyes and get comfortable, taking a few deep breaths to ground yourself. As you do so, start picturing the outcome or practice you want. Suppose that you're visualizing the fit and fabulous future you have. Try to imagine this future self in as much detail as you can. Don't just focus on the visual details, either. Try to imagine and feel how strong your muscles, bones, and body have become. Try to feel how much more stamina and endurance you have, how your reach has increased, how much more flexible you've become, how you can move about a lot more freely, and how much more energy you have now that you've become as fit as you wanted to be (Mind Tools Content Team, 2023).

Alternatively, envision the workout you're about to undertake, particularly on days and moments you don't feel like working out. Mentally walk through your workout routine, and be sure to include even your rest times in this process. Be as detailed as you can as you imagine this workout session. Again, don't just focus on the visual details. Focus on how your muscles will burn as you execute one move. Try to feel how your breathing rate will pick up as you exercise. Try to imagine the sounds you'll hear around you as you work, how the temperature of the room will fluctuate as you physically exert yourself, to feel the breeze if you imagine yourself on the run, or how your steps will pound the ground or treadmill if that's what you're envisioning yourself on.

By doing these two visualization exercises, you'll achieve two things. First, you'll increase your motivation that day to follow through with your workout plan. Second, you'll mentally prime yourself to work out by tricking your mind into believing you already are. Thus, you'll overcome any resistance you have to the practice.

## Long-Term Fitness and Health Habits

Once you've begun your fitness journey, you want to take steps that will allow you to adopt fitness and health habits that will last you a lifetime. The first such habit you want to adopt—and say it with me—is con-sis-ten-cy. If you want to make health and fitness into permanent parts of your life, you have to *commit* to it. You have to consistently work out and maintain a healthy diet. That's not to say you can't have rest days or even cheat days. In fact, you should most definitely have rest days to give your body the time it needs to recover from your arduous exercise sessions. You can also have cheat days. I mean, what's a birthday without a slice of cake? Notice that I've said a "slice," though, meaning that you should take care not to overdo it. You should also ensure those cheat days don't turn into cheat weeks or cheat months.

Once you've made this commitment, SMART goal-setting will be your best friend. Regularly go over your daily, weekly, and even monthly fitness goals. Keep track of the ones you achieve and keep your motivation and commitment levels high. If you notice that a goal you've set for yourself is just a little out of the realm of possibility for you for that given moment, then be flexible enough to adjust it. Also, be kind to yourself if you have an occasional off day, which you will do. Some days, working out will be a little harder than others; some days, your performance will not match that of the previous one. That's perfectly alright and to be expected. Remind yourself of that. Also, remind yourself that there will be days when you perform better than expected, and you have to keep going to have those days, just as you have to keep going to achieve the health and fitness level that you want (*Healthy Habits for Long-Term Fitness Success*, 2024).

That being said, try listening to and understanding your body throughout this process. Your body gives you clear signs about what it needs. All you need to do to hear them is to listen. For example, if you've hit an exercise plateau, as discussed before, that's probably your body telling you that you need to change things up. If you're feeling really jittery these days, then that's likely your body telling you it needs more movement and effort. If, on the other hand, your body feels more achy than usual and tired, that's most likely a sign that you can and should take an extra rest day and maybe make some adjustments to your diet. If the situation persists for a few days, then it might be that you're getting sick. So, resting a few extra days, monitoring the situation, and going to the doctor, if need be, is a good idea.

A final step you need to take to adopt healthy and lifelong lifestyle habits is to understand how new habits are formed and then leverage that process to adopt the habits you want in life. Habits are formed through two processes. First, when you start a new habit, neural pathways—meaning connections between various brain cells—form in your brain; these neural pathways are used each time you perform the actions associated with a given movement. Each time you repeat those actions, the neural pathways linked to them become stronger. If those pathways become strong enough, then the actions they're associated with become automatic. Thus, habits are formed, and you don't even have to think about them to do them.

Second, habits follow a typical three-step cycle (Gardner et al., 2012):

1. The habit cue

2. The routine

3. The reward

Let's assume that you have a habit of eating junk food whenever you feel stressed. Your habit starts when something happens that triggers your stress response, making you open the box of chocolates you keep in the kitchen cupboard. This is your habit cue, which signals that you should begin said habit. The routine is the act of eating and finishing the entire box in one sitting. The reward is the flood of endorphins that are released in your system as a result of these actions. Since endorphins are feel-good hormones, the real reward here is the stress relief that eating that box of chocolates provides you. Here's the issue: The stress relief that that box of chocolate will provide you with will be temporary. You'll feel stressed again in no time at all and want to reach for another box of chocolates. Add to that how unhealthy eating a box or two of chocolates in one go will be for you, and it's easy to see why this is a problematic habit.

What if you wanted to replace this habit? In this case, you'd have to identify what reward you're seeking through this habit. That reward is stress relief, as we said. So, you can choose a habit that'll give you this same reward but will be better for your health in the long run. This will make it easier for you to let go of an unhealthy habit and commit to a new, healthy one instead. What habits provide you with stress relief? Off the top of my head, there's meditation and exercise. Let's say you've decided to adopt meditation as a replacement habit. How do you go about doing that?

Start by determining what your habit cue will be and try to make it similar to the cue of your original, unhealthy habit. Your habit cue for the chocolate habit recognizes that you're getting stressed. Your habit cue for meditation will be the same. Your routine for this habit, however, will be different. Instead of opening the kitchen cupboard and reaching for the chocolates, you'll open your bedroom door, turn on some relaxing music, and sit down on a comfortable surface to start meditation, as described in previous chapters. At first, your body will show a little resistance to this, craving the immediate satisfaction the chocolates will provide over the one meditation since the latter will take a little while longer to kick in. Focus on your meditation when this happens. Allow your craving thoughts to drift in and out of your mind as they please. Believe me, after a little while, they will drift away, so long as you don't go chasing after them. Remember to focus on your breath and the moment you're in if you're struggling. After a short while, those thoughts will subside, and your stress response will start calming down, too, allowing you to achieve the reward you were seeking in the first place.

# Conclusion

We may be at the end of this book, but we're also at the very beginning of your journey. Reading *Fit and Proud* was your first step in starting your fitness and health adventure as you head into your 50s and beyond. Now, you need to take the many other steps we've covered and actually put what you have learned into practice. In other words, you need to make a commitment, here and now, to live the best possible life you can and start taking conscious action to do so. What does this process entail? Let's quickly review what we've learned throughout *Fit and Proud* to answer this question. Throughout the course of this book, we have covered the following topics:

- We explored the physical and mental changes that come with aging to better understand what happens to us as we age. We also discussed what unique challenges gay men over 55 personally experience in this regard.

- We discussed how we can set fitness goals that are right for both our age and our current fitness level, create a sustainable fitness plan that works for us, and track our progress as we make headway.

- We came to understand the nutritional needs of our aging minds and bodies, what we need to consume to meet those needs, and how we can maintain a healthy, balanced, and tasty diet. Similarly, we took into account any chronic diseases we may have as we plan our diet.

- We went over how important strength training is for us as we age, how we can safely perform strength training exercises, and which resistance training exercises are best for us in our 50s (and beyond).

- We also delved into the importance of doing cardio and what kind of exercises we must adopt to maintain our health and well-being. Here, we covered various tips that can help us to improve our stamina and endurance levels.

- We talked about what a healthy body composition looks like at 55, why this is important, and what activities and habits we need to embrace so that we can ensure we have healthy body compositions ourselves.

- We covered the wide variety of flexibility, mobility, and balance exercises we can do in light of the fact that our joints and muscles become less flexible as we age and the fact that our balance gets a bit wonky over time, thereby increasing our risk of falling and injuring ourselves.

- We delved into the importance of looking after our sexual health as we age (since we don't magically become celibate monks once we hit 50) and what we need to do to keep maintaining it.

- We've seen what mindfulness and mental health practices we should adopt to strengthen and improve our mental health and how we can incorporate them into our daily lives and routines.

- We grasped how vital strong support systems and social lives are as we age, especially for us as members of the LGBTQ+ community, and how we can improve our relationships and forge new, healthy ones with our community.

- We went through the various barriers we might have when working out and the different techniques we can adopt to overcome them. We also introduced strategies that will help us should we relapse, for lack of a better word.

- We explored the numerous strategies, techniques, and methods we can embrace to adopt healthy lifestyle habits, making them permanent.

When you look at it like that, we have really covered a great deal throughout the course of this book. Now is the time to roll up your sleeves and get to work so that you can transform your life and your health in the way you want. With all that said, there's really only one question left to ask: Are you ready to begin?

# Exercise Sheets

Since developing a solid routine and keeping track of your progress is immeasurably important when it comes to exercising, here are some bonus exercise sheets to help you do just that:

| DATE | | TRAINING : | | | | | |
|---|---|---|---|---|---|---|---|
| | S M T W T F S | | | | | | |
| EXERCISE TYPE | | SET 1 | SET 2 | SET 3 | SET 4 | SET 5 | SET 6 |
| 1 | WEIGHT | | | | | | |
| | REPS | | | | | | |
| 2 | | | | | | | |
| 3 | | | | | | | |
| 4 | | | | | | | |
| 5 | | | | | | | |
| 6 | | | | | | | |
| 7 | | | | | | | |
| 8 | | | | | | | |
| 9 | | | | | | | |
| 10 | | | | | | | |
| 11 | | | | | | | |

| CARDIO TYPE | LEVEL | TIME | KCALs |
|---|---|---|---|
| | | | |
| | | | |
| | | | |
| | | | |

| NOTES | SESSION RATING |
|---|---|
| | — |

DATE _____    TRAINING : _____

S M T W T F S

| EXERCISE TYPE | | SET 1 | SET 2 | SET 3 | SET 4 | SET 5 | SET 6 |
|---|---|---|---|---|---|---|---|
| 1 | WEIGHT | | | | | | |
| | REPS | | | | | | |
| 2 | | | | | | | |
| 3 | | | | | | | |
| 4 | | | | | | | |
| 5 | | | | | | | |
| 6 | | | | | | | |
| 7 | | | | | | | |
| 8 | | | | | | | |
| 9 | | | | | | | |
| 10 | | | | | | | |
| 11 | | | | | | | |

| CARDIO TYPE | LEVEL | TIME | KCALs |
|---|---|---|---|
| | | | |
| | | | |
| | | | |
| | | | |

| NOTES | SESSION RATING |
|---|---|
| | _____ |

DATE _____ TRAINING : _____

S M T W T F S

| EXERCISE TYPE | | SET 1 | SET 2 | SET 3 | SET 4 | SET 5 | SET 6 |
|---|---|---|---|---|---|---|---|
| 1 | WEIGHT | | | | | | |
| | REPS | | | | | | |
| 2 | | | | | | | |
| 3 | | | | | | | |
| 4 | | | | | | | |
| 5 | | | | | | | |
| 6 | | | | | | | |
| 7 | | | | | | | |
| 8 | | | | | | | |
| 9 | | | | | | | |
| 10 | | | | | | | |
| 11 | | | | | | | |

| CARDIO TYPE | LEVEL | TIME | KCALs |
|---|---|---|---|
| | | | |
| | | | |
| | | | |
| | | | |

| NOTES | SESSION RATING |
|---|---|
| | ____ |

# Glossary

**Adrenalin:** A hormone that gets released in your body that gets your heart beating really fast in response to rising stress levels.

**Ageism:** The prejudice or discrimination shown against someone because of their age.

**AIDS:** A disease that is caused by the human immunodeficiency virus (HIV) that weakens the immune system, putting people at an increased risk of catching an infection or developing certain types of cancer.

**Alzheimer's:** A brain disorder that sometimes happens with age where the patient slowly loses their memory and thinking skills, ultimately becoming unable to carry out even the simplest of tasks.

**Anxiety:** A disorder where you experience feelings of dread, uneasiness, and fear regularly.

**Body composition:** The overall percentage of muscle, bone, and fat that your body is made up of.

**Body mass index (BMI):** The figure obtained by dividing your weight in kilograms by your height squared, which indicates your physical fitness and health level.

**Bone density:** The measure of your bones' mineral content and how dense or not they are, indicating how strong or not your bones are overall.

**Carbohydrates:** The sugar molecules that are found in certain types of food and that serve as your body's main source of energy.

**Cardiovascular system:** Your body's circulatory system, which is made up of your heart, veins, and your lungs, seeing as your lungs pump oxygen into your blood.

**Cells:** The smallest organic compound that your body and all your organs and systems are made up of.

**Cholesterol:** A fat-like, waxy substance that's produced by the liver and is found in the bloodstream.

**Community:** A group of individuals that subscribe to the same values, norms, customs, or belief systems that offer one another support and a sense of belonging.

**Cortisol:** A hormone that is released in your body whenever your stress response is triggered, causing you to display the classic signs of stress, including tensing muscles and a rapid heartbeat.

**Depression:** A pervasive feeling of sadness that you can't seem to get away from and a loss of interest in activities you ordinarily enjoy.

**Diet:** The meals that you regularly consume in your daily life and the meal plan you follow.

**Discrimination:** The unjust or prejudicial behaviors shown to different groups of people simply on account of their differences.

**Emotional Health:** Our sense of general well-being based on how we feel and think.

**Endorphin:** A kind of hormone that is released within your body that makes you feel good and whose release is triggered by you doing pleasurable activities such as working out, getting a massage, having sex, or doing an activity you otherwise enjoy.

**Endurance:** Your body's ability to withstand physical exertion and stress.

**Fats:** The nutrients found in certain foods that your body uses to build cells' membranes, nerve tissues, and hormones.

**Flexibility:** Your joints' ability to move freely without any restrictions or pain.

**Heart disease:** A range of disorders and conditions that negatively affect the heart, such as a heart attack or coronary heart disease.

**Heart Rate:** The number of times your heart beats per minute, which is subject to change depending on your level of exertion at the time.

**HIIT:** High intensity interval training, where you put your body through really intense exercises for short bursts of time to get your blood pumping.

**HIV:** A virus that attacks the body's own immune system, thereby weakening it to the point that it becomes incapable of fighting off illnesses.

**Hormone:** Chemical messengers that your brain sends throughout your body, giving various systems and organs orders to do different things, like tense your muscles if you're stressed and the hormone in question is a stress hormone, or relax your muscles if the hormone in question is a feel-good hormone.

**Interval Training:** A series of high intensity trainings that are broken up by short rest periods.

**Meditation:** A mindfulness practice where you concentrate on your breathing and on clearing your mind through the use of various relaxation techniques and mental techniques.

**Mental Health:** Your overall emotional, psychological, and social well-being, which allows you to manage your stress levels, relate to other people, and make sound decisions in life.

**Metabolism:** The chemical process that happens within your body to convert the food you eat into energy your body can use to perform the daily tasks you're going to perform.

**Mobility:** Your ability to move about freely and unrestricted without experiencing any pain.

**Muscle Mass:** The overall muscle weight within your body in pounds or kilograms.

**Nerves:** A bundle of fibers that run through the spinal cord and connect to different parts of your body, allowing your brain to set orders for it so that you can perform the tasks you need to perform.

**Neural pathway:** The connections that form between different brain cells, allowing you to perform different sets of tasks.

**Neurodegenerative condition:** A condition or disease where your brain cells and the cells making up your nervous system lose their functions over time and start dying off.

**Neuron:** The cells making up your brain and nervous system.

**Nervous system:** The system in your body that is made up of your spinal cord, brain, and the network of nerves that run through your body, allowing your brain to send messages to the rest of your body so that it can perform the tasks it needs to perform.

**Nutrition:** Supplying the various organic and non-organic components that make up the food you eat, such as vitamins and minerals, that your body needs to function properly.

**Osteoporosis:** An aging-related condition where the density and thickness of your bone tissue decrease as time goes by, causing your bones to become weaker and, therefore, easier to break.

**Pacemaker cells:** Very specialized cells in your heart that dictate your regular, stress-free heartbeat.

**Pilates:** A low-intensity exercise that strengthens your muscles and increases your flexibility while improving your posture and mobility.

**PrEP:** The medicine you take to keep from getting HIV.

**Protein:** The main molecule that meat products are made of, which your body needs to build muscle and knit together other things like hair, skin tissue, and enzymes.

**Self-acceptance:** Your ability to accept yourself as you are, flaws and all, while committing to improve upon your strengths.

**Self-care:** Activities that allow you to rest and recover, such as meditation, sleep, and journaling, that take care of your physical, mental, and emotional health.

**Self-compassion:** The kindness and love you show yourself through your actions, words, and thoughts.

**Self-love:** The love you show yourself by practicing self-care, self-acceptance, and self-compassion.

**Social support:** The help the people in your life give you, particularly the individuals in your social system, when you need it.

**Stamina:** Your body's ability to withstand stress and exertion for extended periods of time.

**Stress:** A state of mental tension and worry caused by a threat or otherwise challenging situation.

**Stress Response:** The chemical and physical your brain and body respectively give to a threatening situation, be it a predator or taxes, getting you ready to fight said threat or flee from it.

**Support network:** The system you create that is made up of people who care about you and offer you support when you need it. You do the same for them in turn.

**Vitamin:** A nutrient that's found in various fruits and vegetables and that comes in different varieties, which your body needs to be able to function properly.

**Yoga:** A low intensity exercise that's been around for centuries that seriously increases your body's flexibility and balance, along with your muscular strength.

# References

Abbate, E. (2019, May 2). *What your body composition metrics actually say about your health.* Men's Health. https://www.menshealth.com/health/a27242669/what-your-body-composition-metrics-say-about-your-health/

*About sleep.* (2024, April 2). U.S. Centers for Disease Control and Prevention. https://www.cdc.gov/sleep/about/

Achauer, H. (2022, December 9). Can you pass the flexibility test? *The New York Times.* https://www.nytimes.com/2022/12/09/well/move/flexibility-test-mobility-fitness.html

Age-related hearing loss (presbycusis) — causes and treatment. (2015, August 18). NIDCD. https://www.nidcd.nih.gov/health/age-related-hearing-loss#:~:text=It%20is%20one%20of%20the

American Heart Association Staff. (2018, April 18). *Breaking down barriers to fitness.* American Heart Association. https://www.heart.org/en/healthy-living/fitness/getting-active/breaking-down-barriers-to-fitness

*Aquatic exercise: number of participants U.S. 2018.* (2019). Statista. https://www.statista.com/statistics/191380/participants-in-aquatic-exercise-in-the-us-since-2006/

Asher, A. (2015, August 12). *7 great hamstring stretches.* Verywell Health. https://www.verywellhealth.com/great-hamstring-stretches-296849

Asp, K. (2024, April 2). *Are you fit for your age? What really counts.* WebMD. https://www.webmd.com/fitness-exercise/features/fit-for-your-age

Barone, L. (2024, January 24). *Breaking down barriers to exercise as we get older.* Elossa Fitness. https://elossafitness.com/breaking-down-barriers-to-exercise-as-we-get-older/

*Benefits of LGBTQIA+ team sports and group exercise.* (2024, April 15). UPMC HealthBeat. https://share.upmc.com/2024/04/lgbtqia-team-sports/

Bertoia, M. L., Mukamal, K. J., Cahill, L. E., Hou, T., Ludwig, D. S., Mozaffarian, D., Willett, W. C., Hu, F. B., & Rimm, E. B. (2015). Changes in Intake of Fruits and Vegetables and Weight Change in United States Men and Women Followed for Up to 24 Years: Analysis from Three Prospective Cohort Studies. *PLOS Medicine,* *12*(9), e1001878. https://doi.org/10.1371/journal.pmed.1001878

Better Health Channel Staff. (2012). *Physical activity - staying motivated.* Better Health Channel. https://www.betterhealth.vic.gov.au/health/healthyliving/physical-activity-staying-motivated

Bowen, V. (2023). *Maintaining flexibility with aging.* Arthritis and Rheumatism Associates, P.C. https://arapc.com/maintaining-flexibility-with-aging/#:~:text=As%20our%20bodies%20get%20older

Brennan, D. (2021a, October 18). *Best dynamic stretches for older adults.* WebMD. https://www.webmd.com/healthy-aging/9-best-dynamic-stretches-for-older-adults

Brennan, D. (2021b, October 25). *What to know about emotional health.* WebMD. https://www.webmd.com/balance/what-to-know-about-emotional-health

Brennan, D. (2021c, November 1). *What to know about mental health in older adults.* WebMD. https://www.webmd.com/healthy-aging/mental-health-in-older-adults

Brett, M. (2023, November 7). *How to boost your cycling fitness when you're aged over 50.* Road Cycling.

https://road.cc/content/feature/how-boost-your-fitness-
when-youre-aged-over-50-304835

Brixius, K. (2022, March 22). *How to track your fitness progress.* Nutrisense
Journal. https://www.nutrisense.io/blog/how-to-track-your-
fitness

Brown, K. (2023, June 22). Does working out increase sex drive? Hims.
https://www.hims.com/blog/working-out-increase-sex-drive

*Calf stretch.* (n.d.). Mayo Clinic. https://www.mayoclinic.org/diseases-
conditions/muscle-cramp/multimedia/calf-stretch/img-
20007902

Carter, S. (2022, October 22). *Why it's important to cool down after exercise,
according to the science.* Live Science.
https://www.livescience.com/why-its-important-to-cool-
down-after-exercise-according-to-the-science

Cassata, C. (2021, September 25). *Flaws and all: How to accept yourself in 8
steps.* Psych Central. https://psychcentral.com/lib/ways-to-
accept-yourself

Celias. (2023, September 15). *The importance of lifelong learning as you age.*
Vista Grande Villa. https://vistagrandevilla.com/the-
importance-of-lifelong-learning-as-you-
age/#:~:text=Supports%20brain%20health.&text=Research%
20shows%20that%20lifelong%20learners

Chen, M. A. (2022, August 16). *Being active when you have heart disease.*
MedlinePlus Medical Encyclopedia.
https://medlineplus.gov/ency/patientinstructions/000094.htm
#:~:text=Expand%20Section-

Cherney, K. (2022, September 19). *Effects of anxiety on the body.*
Healthline.
https://www.healthline.com/health/anxiety/effects-on-
body#immune

Cherry, K. (2023, March 3). *How social support contributes to psychological health*. Verywell Mind. https://www.verywellmind.com/social-support-for-psychological-health-4119970

Chopik, W. J., Bremner, R. H., Johnson, D. J., & Giasson, H. L. (2018). Age Differences in Age Perceptions and Developmental Transitions. *Frontiers in Psychology, 9*(1). https://doi.org/10.3389/fpsyg.2018.00067

Cleveland Clinic Staff. (2021, August 16). *How box breathing can help you destress*. Cleveland Clinic. https://health.clevelandclinic.org/box-breathing-benefits

Cleveland Clinic Staff. (2024, January 4). *6 reasons mental health is so important*. Cleveland Clinic. https://health.clevelandclinic.org/why-mental-health-is-so-important

Contributors, W. E. (2022, November 29). *7 tips for better sex after 50*. WebMD. https://www.webmd.com/healthy-aging/sex-after-50

Cooks-Campbell, A. (2022, May 26). *What self-love truly means and ways to cultivate it*. BetterUp. https://www.betterup.com/blog/self-love

*Coping with stress*. (2023, April 28). U.S. Centers for Disease Control and Prevention. https://www.cdc.gov/mentalhealth/cope-with-stress/

Craig, H. (2019, March 4). *10 ways to build trust in a relationship*. Positive Psychology. https://positivepsychology.com/build-trust/#build-trust

Crichton-Stuart, C. (2020, November 26). *The top 10 benefits of eating healthy*. Medical News Today. https://www.medicalnewstoday.com/articles/322268#better-sleep

Cronkleton, E. (2019, July 29). *How and when to include static stretching in your workout*. Healthline.

https://www.healthline.com/health/exercise-fitness/static-stretching#examples

Cronkleton, E. (2022, April 29). *6 ways to bust through a workout plateau.* Healthline. https://www.healthline.com/nutrition/workout-plateau#how-to-break-it

Crouch, M. (2024, May 29). *Top exercise for brain and body.* AARP. https://www.aarp.org/health/healthy-living/info-2024/tai-chi-benefits.html#:~:text=1%20exercise%20for%20an%20aging

Davidson, K. (2021, September 20). *The definitive guide to healthy eating in your 50s and 60s.* Healthline. https://www.healthline.com/nutrition/healthy-eating-50s-60s#nutrients-foods

Dawn Neumann, K. (2016, July 18). *Proper squat form 101 and how to squat effectively.* Real Simple. https://www.realsimple.com/health/fitness-exercise/workouts/squat-form

*Discover 7 surprising health benefits of swimming over 50.* (2023, June 6). Simply Swim UK. https://www.simplyswim.com/blogs/blog/discover-7-surprising-health-benefits-of-swimming-over-50

Easter, M. (2019, September 25). *What to know before starting intermittent fasting.* Men's Health. https://www.menshealth.com/nutrition/a29192545/intermittent-fasting-beginners-guide/

Editors of Men's Health. (2021, January 1). *4 steps to staying fit after 50.* Men's Health. https://www.menshealth.com/fitness/a35091902/men-over-50-workout-tips/

Edwards, T. (2022, April 1). *How to build muscle strength: A complete guide.* Healthline. https://www.healthline.com/health/fitness/how-to-build-strength-guide#tips

*Exercise for heart failure: tips for exercising safely.* (2022, June). Britihs Heart Foundation. https://www.bhf.org.uk/informationsupport/heart-matters-magazine/activity/exercise-for-heart-failure#:~:text=It

*Facts about falls.* (2024, June 10). Centers for Disease Control and Prevention. https://www.cdc.gov/falls/data-research/facts-stats/index.html#:~:text=In%20fact%2C%20more%20than%20one

*Fat intake calculator.* (n.d.). Calculator. Retrieved June 4, 2024, from https://www.calculator.net/fat-intake-calculator.html?cage=55&csex=m&cheightfeet=5&cheightinch=10&cpound=160&cheightmeter=180&ckg=60&cactivity=1.375&cmop=0&cformula=m&cfatpct=20&printit=0&ctype=metric&x=Calculate

Felman, A. (2020, April 13). *Mental health: Definition, common disorders, and early signs.* Medical News Today. https://www.medicalnewstoday.com/articles/154543#definition

*5 tips for improving physical stamina in your 50s.* (2022, January 5). TerraBella Senior Living. https://www.terrabellaseniorliving.com/senior-living-blog/5-tips-for-improving-physical-stamina-in-your-50s/

Fletcher, J. (2019, August 22). *6 essential nutrients: Sources and why you need them.* Medical News Today. https://www.medicalnewstoday.com/articles/326132#water

*Foam rolling for 50+.* (2019, May 21). Life Enriching Communities. https://lec.org/blog/health/foam-rolling-for-50/

*Foods high in potassium.* (2021, June 2). Healthdirect Australia. https://www.healthdirect.gov.au/foods-high-in-potassium

Frazier, R. S. (2021, November 15). *You're almost definitely not getting enough sleep.* Men's Health.

https://www.menshealth.com/health/a38113961/how-much-sleep-do-you-need-every-night/

Fredriksen-Goldsen, K. I. (2011). Resilience and disparities among lesbian, gay, bisexual, and transgender older adults. *Public Policy & Aging Report, 21*(3), 3–7. https://doi.org/10.1093/ppar/21.3.3

Gardner, B., Lally, P., & Wardle, J. (2012). Making health habitual: the psychology of "habit-formation" and general practice. *British Journal of General Practice, 62*(605), 664–666. https://doi.org/10.3399/bjgp12x659466

Gainer, L. (2023, May 23). *7 ways to build a social support system for better health.* Well Theory. https://www.welltheory.com/resources/7-ways-to-build-a-social-support-system-for-better-health

Gidus, T. (2011, January 13). *Healthy eating for seniors.* Healthline. https://www.healthline.com/health/healthy-eating-for-seniors#age-related-changes

Godman, H. (2022, July 1). *Use strength training to help ward off chronic disease.* Harvard Health. https://www.health.harvard.edu/staying-healthy/use-strength-training-to-help-ward-off-chronic-disease

Harvard Health Publishing Staff. (2018, August 1). *How meditation helps with depression.* Harvard Health. https://www.health.harvard.edu/mind-and-mood/how-meditation-helps-with-depression

Healthline Editorial Team. (2022, February 17). *Stress and anxiety: How they differ and how to manage them.* Healthline. https://www.healthline.com/health/stress-and-anxiety#coping-tips

*Healthy eating over 60.* (2020, February 10). Healthdirect Australia. https://www.healthdirect.gov.au/healthy-eating-over-60

*Healthy habits for long-term fitness success.* (2024, May 10). Genetic Nutrition. https://www.geneticnutrition.in/blogs/genetic-life/healthy-habits-for-long-term-fitness-success#:~:text=Building%20a%20routine%20that%20includes

Hernandez, M. (2023, April 26). *Benefits of having a fitness community*. Chuze Fitness. https://chuzefitness.com/blog/benefits-of-having-a-fitness-community/

*Healthy habits for long-term fitness success*. (2024, May 10). Genetic Nutrition. https://www.geneticnutrition.in/blogs/genetic-life/healthy-habits-for-long-term-fitness-success#:~:text=Building%20a%20routine%20that%20includes

*How does sleep reduce stress?* (n.d.). Everlywell: Home Health Testing Made Easy. https://www.everlywell.com/blog/sleep-and-stress/how-does-sleep-reduce-stress/#sleep-stress-cycle

*How to work out smarter, not harder*. (2022, November 16). Cleveland Clinic. https://health.clevelandclinic.org/smart-fitness-goals

*The importance of rest*. (2023, May 19). Auckland Physiotherapy. https://www.aucklandphysiotherapy.co.nz/blog/the-importance-of-rest/#:~:text=By%20allowing%20our%20bodies%20time

Jimenez, M. P. (2021). Associations between Nature Exposure and Health: a Review of the Evidence. *International Journal of Environmental Research and Public Health*, *18*(9), 4790. https://doi.org/10.3390/ijerph18094790

Kandola, A. (2019, May 14). *Simple carbs vs. complex carbs: What's the difference?* Medical News Today. https://www.medicalnewstoday.com/articles/325171#:~:text=Complex%20carbohydrates%20take%20longer%20to

Kendrick, G. (2023, January 4). *Attainable fitness goals for older adults*. Prestige Care. https://www.prestigecare.com/blog/attainable-fitness-goals-for-older-adults/

Lennon, A. (2020, December 15). *Why it's still important for seniors to set goals.* CarePatrol. https://carepatrol.com/blog/why-its-still-important-for-seniors-to-set-goals/#:~:text=By%20setting%20short%2Dterm%20goals

Liu, X., Li, Y., Guasch-Ferré, M., Willett, W. C., Drouin-Chartier, J.-P., Bhupathiraju, S. N., & Tobias, D. K. (2019). Changes in nut consumption influence long-term weight change in US men and women. *BMJ Nutrition, Prevention & Health*, *2*(2), 90–99. https://doi.org/10.1136/bmjnph-2019-000034

Llyod, D. (n.d.). *9 easy ways to get started with yoga over 50.* David Llyod Blog. https://blog.davidlloyd.co.uk/exercise-classes/yoga-over-50/#:~:text=There's%20no%20maximum%20age%20%E2%80%93%20you,with%20breathwork%20and%20some%20meditation.

Luff, C. (2022, May 28). *8 tips for running in your 40s, 50s, and beyond.* Verywell Fit. https://www.verywellfit.com/tips-for-running-in-your-50s-and-beyond-2911208

MacDonald , M. (2024, April 2). *Bend, don't break: Flexibility training tips for the over-50s.* Dr. MacDonald Cardiologist. https://heartdoctormacdonald.com/bend-dont-break-flexibility-training-tips-for-the-over-50s/

Madison. (2021, January 18). *How to manage balance problems in seniors.* MeetCaregivers. https://meetcaregivers.com/balance-problems-in-seniors/#:~:text=Balance%20problems%20in%20seniors%20often

Mayo Clinic Staff. (2017a). *Measure your fitness level with these simple tests.* Mayo Clinic. https://www.mayoclinic.org/healthy-lifestyle/fitness/in-depth/fitness/art-20046433

Mayo Clinic Staff. (2017b). *Senior sex: What older men want to know.* Mayo Clinic. https://www.mayoclinic.org/healthy-lifestyle/sexual-health/in-depth/senior-sex/art-20046465

Mayo Clinic Staff. (2022, August 3). *Exercise and stress: Get moving to manage stress.* Mayo Clinic. https://www.mayoclinic.org/healthy-lifestyle/stress-management/in-depth/exercise-and-stress/art-20044469

McCoy, J. (2016, March 24). *How to start working out again when it's been awhile.* Self. https://www.self.com/story/heres-exactly-how-to-ease-back-into-working-out

Mellardo, A. (2022, October 21). *What a daily walking habit does to your body after 50, says science.* Eat This Not That. https://www.eatthis.com/what-daily-walking-does-to-your-body-after-50/

Menzies, R. (2021, October 12). *Pilates for seniors: Benefits, considerations, and more.* Healthline. https://www.healthline.com/health/fitness/pilates-for-seniors#considerations

Mind Tools Content Team. (2023). *Visualization.* MindTools. https://www.mindtools.com/a5ycdws/visualization

National Institute on Aging Staff. (2020). *10 myths about aging.* National Institute on Aging. https://www.nia.nih.gov/health/10-myths-about-aging

Nazario, B. (2023). *What's normal (and what's not) as you age.* WebMD. https://www.webmd.com/healthy-aging/story/what-to-expect-aging

Painter, J. A., Elliott, S. J., & Hudson, S. (2009). Falls in community-dwelling adults aged 50 years and older: prevalence and contributing factors. *Journal of Allied Health, 38*(4), 201–207. https://pubmed.ncbi.nlm.nih.gov/20011818/

Pierce-Smith, D., & Watson, L. R. (n.d.). *Screening guidelines for men 50 to 64.* Health Encyclopedia - University of Rochester Medical Center. https://www.urmc.rochester.edu/encyclopedia/content.aspx?contenttypeid=43&contentid=men5064

Ratini, M. (2024, February 29). *What to know about cardio for men over fifty*. WebMD. https://www.webmd.com/healthy-aging/what-to-know-cardio-men-over-fifty

Raypole, C. (2020, September 1). *Do affirmations work? Yes, but there's a catch*. Healthline. https://www.healthline.com/health/mental-health/do-affirmations-work

Reblin, M., & Uchino, B. N. (2018). Social and emotional support and its implication for health. *Current Opinion in Psychiatry, 21*(2), 201–205. https://doi.org/10.1097/yco.0b013e3282f3ad89

Ritchey, C. (2023, May 22). *Here's what you need to know about weight training for weight loss*. Men's Health. https://www.menshealth.com/weight-loss/a43760101/weight-training-for-weight-loss/

Rogers, P. (2022, July 29). *Dumbbell overhead press workout for the shoulders and triceps*. Verywell Fit. https://www.verywellfit.com/how-to-do-the-dumbbell-overhead-press-3498298

Rowan, G. A., Frimpong, E. Y., Li, M., Chaudhry, S., & Radigan, M. (2021). Health Disparities Between Older Lesbian, Gay, and Bisexual Adults and Heterosexual Adults in the Public Mental Health System. *Psychiatric Services*, appi.ps.2020009. https://doi.org/10.1176/appi.ps.202000940

Schroeder, E. C., Franke, W. D., Sharp, R. L., & Lee, D. (2019). Comparative effectiveness of aerobic, resistance, and combined training on cardiovascular disease risk factors: A randomized controlled trial. *PLOS ONE, 14*(1), e0210292. https://doi.org/10.1371/journal.pone.0210292

Scott, E. (2018, February 5). *The benefits of meditation for stress management*. Verywell Mind. https://www.verywellmind.com/meditation-4157199

Scott, E. (2023, October 23). *Is journaling an effective stress management tool?* Verywell Mind. https://www.verywellmind.com/the-benefits-of-journaling-for-stress-management-3144611#toc-strategies-to-try

*Sexuality and aging: Your guide to maintaining sexual health.* (n.d.). Everlywell: Home Health Testing Made Easy. https://www.everlywell.com/blog/sti-testing/sexuality-and-aging/#change

Shetty, M. (2024, January 23). *Protein needs for adults 50+*. Lifestyle Medicine. https://longevity.stanford.edu/lifestyle/2024/01/23/protein-needs-for-adults-50/#:~:text=To%20build%20muscle%20past%20the

Siu, P. M., Yu, A. P., Benzie, I. F., & Woo, J. (2015). Effects of 1-year yoga on cardiovascular risk factors in middle-aged and older adults with metabolic syndrome: a randomized trial. *Diabetology & Metabolic Syndrome*, *7*(1). https://doi.org/10.1186/s13098-015-0034-3

Stanborough, R. J. (2020, February 4). *How to change negative thinking with cognitive restructuring*. Healthline. https://www.healthline.com/health/cognitive-restructuring

Statchel, J. (2023, November 26). *How to boost libido and increase sex drive*. Everlywell: Home Health Testing Made Easy. https://www.everlywell.com/blog/testosterone/boosting-sex-drive/#increase-libido

Stevens, C. (2023, December 14). *HIIT over 50: A 20-minute, low-impact workout for beginners*. Live Strong. https://www.livestrong.com/article/13721855-hiit-workout-over-50/

Stewart, J., Munson, M., & Blumberg, P. O. (2024, January 11). *The 22 best ways to lose weight after 50*. Men's Health. https://www.menshealth.com/weight-loss/a26555881/losing-weight-after-50/

*10 reasons why dancing after 50 is great, and you should do it!* (2021, August 13). Baila for Life. https://bailaforlife.com/10-reasons-why-you-should-be-dancing-after-50/

*10 resistance band workouts for seniors: 20 minute workout included.* (2023, November 10). LIT Method. https://www.litmethod.com/blogs/boltcut-blog/resistance-band-exercises-for-seniors

*13 benefits of strength training for people older than 50.* (n.d.). Human Kinetics Canada. https://canada.humankinetics.com/blogs/articles/13-benefits-of-strength-training-for-people-older-than-50

Tracy, B. L. (n.d.). *Mobility.* Center for Healthy Aging. Retrieved June 11, 2024, from https://www.research.colostate.edu/healthyagingcenter/aging-basics/mobility/#:~:text=Aging%20deteriorates%20neurons%20and%20muscle.&text=Neurons%20are%20lost%20over%20the

Waehner, P. (2019). *Why you should add cardio to your workout routine.* Verywell Fit. https://www.verywellfit.com/everything-you-need-to-know-about-cardio-1229553

Waehner, P. (2022, February 12). *3 sample workout schedules for a complete exercise program.* Verywell Fit. https://www.verywellfit.com/sample-workout-schedule-1230758

Walters, A. (2024, May 18). Brett is the only bloke in his aqua aerobics class and says more men should give it a go. *ABC News.* https://www.abc.net.au/news/2024-05-18/aqua-aerobics-fitness-classes-popular-with-over-50s/103819940

*What older adults should know about eating bad carbs.* (2021, October 9). Integris Health. https://integrishealth.org/resources/on-your-health/2021/october/what-older-adults-should-know-about-eating-bad-carbs#:~:text=The%20latest%20Dietary%20Guidelines%20for,to%201%2C430%20calories%20from%20carbohydrates.

Wheeler, T. (2023, July 20). *What is body composition?* WebMD. https://www.webmd.com/fitness-exercise/what-is-body-composition

Williams, B. (2018, November 15). *How to bench press the right way.* Men's Health. https://www.menshealth.com/fitness/a25126689/how-to-bench-press/

Wirth, J. (2022, October 25). *The most important nutrients as you age—and where to find them.* Forbes Health. https://www.forbes.com/health/healthy-aging/important-nutrients-as-you-age/

Zane, Z. (2020, January 10). *12 exercises that'll make you better at sex.* Men's Health. https://www.menshealth.com/sex-women/g19541499/exercise-for-better-sex/

Zheng, M., Allman-Farinelli, M., Heitmann, B. L., & Rangan, A. (2015). Substitution of sugar-sweetened beverages with other beverage alternatives: A review of long-term health outcomes. *Journal of the Academy of Nutrition and Dietetics, 115*(5), 767–779. https://doi.org/10.1016/j.jand.2015.01.006

# Image References

Zainuddin A. (n.d.). *Arm Curls.* [Illustration]. Fiverr.

Zainuddin A. (n.d.). *Artboard 8.* [Illustration]. Fiverr.

Zainuddin A. (n.d.). *Butterfly Stretch.* [Illustration]. Fiverr.

Zainuddin A. (n.d.). *Calf Stretch.* [Illustration]. Fiverr.

Zainuddin A. (n.d.). *Chair assisted stretches.* [Illustration]. Fiverr.

Zainuddin A. (n.d.). *Chin down.* [Illustration]. Fiverr.

Zainuddin A. (n.d.). *Deadlift.* [Illustration]. Fiverr.

Zainuddin A. (n.d.). *Downward facing dog.* [Illustration]. Fiverr.

Zainuddin A. (n.d.). *Forward dog.* [Illustration]. Fiverr.

Zainuddin A. (n.d.). *Glute bridge.* [Illustration]. Fiverr.

Zainuddin A. (n.d.). *Lunges with weights.* [Illustration]. Fiverr.

Zainuddin A. (n.d.). *Overhead dumbbell press.* [Illustration]. Fiverr.

Zainuddin A. (n.d.). *Plank.* [Illustration]. Fiverr.

Zainuddin A. (n.d.). *Push up.* [Illustration]. Fiverr.

Zainuddin A. (n.d.). *Sitting shoulder stretch.* [Illustration]. Fiverr.

Zainuddin A. (n.d.). *Sitting up warm up stretching.* [Illustration]. Fiverr.

Zainuddin A. (n.d.). *Squats.* [Illustration]. Fiverr.

Zainuddin A. (n.d.). *Standing barbell rows.* [Illustration]. Fiverr.

Zainuddin A. (n.d.). *Standing quad stretch.* [Illustration]. Fiverr.

Zainuddin A. (n.d.). *Workout sheet.* [Illustration]. Fiverr.